Practice-Based Learning and Improvement:

A Clinical Improvement Action Guide

SECOND EDITION

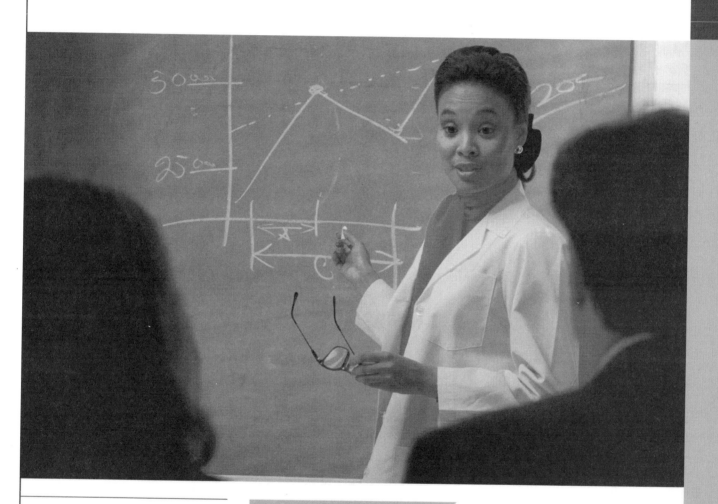

Joint Commission Resources

EDITED BY

Eugene C. Nelson, D.Sc., M.P.H.

Paul B. Batalden, M.D.

Joel S. Lazar, M.D., M.P.H.

Executive Editor: Steven Berman
Project Manager: Cheryl Firestone
Associate Director, Production: Johanna Harris
Executive Director: Catherine Chopp Hinckley, Ph.D.
Vice President, Learning: Charles Macfarlane, F.A.C.H.E.

Joint Commission Resources Mission

The mission of Joint Commission Resources is to continuously improve the safety and quality of care in the United States and in the international community through the provision of education and consultation services and international accreditation.

Joint Commission Resources educational programs and publications support, but are separate from, the accreditation activities of The Joint Commission. Attendees at Joint Commission Resources educational programs and purchasers of Joint Commission Resources publications receive no special consideration or treatment in, or confidential information about, the accreditation process.

Joint Commission Resources, Inc. (JCR), a not-for-profit affiliate of the Joint Commission, has been designated by the Joint Commission to publish publications and multimedia products. JCR reproduces and distributes these materials under license from the Joint Commission.

Printed in the U.S.A. 5 4 3 2 1

Requests for permission to make copies of any part of this work should be mailed to
Permissions Editor
Department of Publications
Joint Commission Resources
One Renaissance Boulevard
Oakbrook Terrace, Illinois 60181
permissions@jcrinc.com

ISBN: 978-1-59940-081-5
Library of Congress Control Number: 2007932538
For more information about Joint Commission Resources, please visit http://www.jcrinc.com.

TABLE OF CONTENTS

CONTRIBUTORS

Paul B. Batalden, M.D., is Professor, Departments of Pediatrics and Community and Family Medicine; Director of Health Care Improvement Leadership Development, Dartmouth Medical School, Hanover, New Hampshire; and Director of Clinical Process Improvement and Leadership Development, Dartmouth-Hitchcock Medical Center, Lebanon, New Hampshire.

Donald M. Berwick, M.D., M.P.P., is President and Chief Executive Officer, Institute for Healthcare Improvement, Cambridge, Massachusetts.

Kenneth P. Brin, M.D, Ph.D., is Director of Cardiology, The Heart Hospital at Geisinger-Wyoming Valley Medical Center, Wilkes-Barre, Pennsylvania.

William H. Edwards, M.D., is Professor and Vice Chair of Pediatrics, Neonatology Division Chief, and Section Chief, Neonatal Intensive Care Unit, Children's Hospital at Dartmouth-Hitchcock Medical Center, Lebanon, New Hampshire.

Tina C. Foster, M.D., M.P.H., M.S., is Associate Program Director, Dartmouth-Hitchcock Leadership Preventive Medicine Residency, and Associate Director, Graduate Medical Education, Dartmouth-Hitchcock Medical Center, Lebanon, New Hampshire; and Associate Professor of Obstetrics and Gynecology and Community and Family Medicine, Dartmouth Medical School, Hanover, New Hampshire.

Marjorie M. Godfrey, M.S., R.N., is Instructor in Community and Family Medicine, Dartmouth Medical School, Hanover, New Hampshire; and a Technical Advisor to the Institute for Healthcare Improvement, the Vermont Oxford Network, and other professional organizations in the United States and abroad.

Brent C. James, M.D., M.Stat., is Vice President for Medical Research and Executive Director, Institute for Health Care Delivery Research, Intermountain Healthcare, Salt Lake City.

Julie K. Johnson, **M.S.P.H., Ph.D.**, is Assistant Professor, Department of Medicine at the University of Chicago School of Medicine, Chicago; and Director of Research, American Board of Medical Specialties, Evanston, Illinois.

Joel S. Lazar, M.D., M.P.H., is Assistant Professor of Community and Family Medicine, Dartmouth Medical School, Hanover, New Hampshire; and Director of Quality Improvement, Dartmouth-Hitchcock Medical Center's Community Health Center, Hanover, New Hampshire.

David C. Leach, M.D., is Executive Director, Accreditation Council for Graduate Medical Education, Chicago.

Christina C. Mahoney, R.N., M.S.N., is Staff Nurse, Inpatient Surgical Services and Intensive Care Unit, York Hospital, York, Maine.

Eugene C. Nelson, D.Sc., M.P.H., is Professor, Department of Community and Family Medicine, Dartmouth Medical School, Hanover, New Hampshire; and Director of Quality Administration, Dartmouth-Hitchcock Medical Center, Lebanon, New Hampshire.

Greg S. Ogrinc, M.D., M.S., is Assistant Dean for Research and Innovation in Medical Education and Assistant Professor of Community and Family Medicine and Medicine, Dartmouth Medical School, Hanover, New Hampshire.

Stephen K. Plume, M.D., is President Emeritus of the Dartmouth-Hitchcock Clinic, Lebanon, New Hampshire; and Professor, Department of Surgery, Dartmouth Medical School, Hanover, New Hampshire.

Jeanne C. Ryer, M.S., is Program Director, Endowment for Health, Concord, New Hampshire, a charitable foundation that serves New Hampshire.

James N. Weinstein, D.O., M.S., is Professor and Chairman, Department of Orthopaedic Surgery, Dartmouth-Hitchcock Medical Center, Lebanon, New Hampshire; and the Director of the Institute for Health Policy and Clinical Practice, Dartmouth Medical School, Hanover, New Hampshire.

Reviewers

The comments and advice of the following reviewers are gratefully acknowledged:

Neil Korsen, M.D., M.S., is Associate Director, Center for Outcomes Research and Evaluation, Maine Medical Center, Portland, Maine.

Karen McKinley, R.N., M.B.A., is Vice President, Clinical Effectiveness, Geisinger Health System, Danville, Pennyslvania.

FOREWORD

Donald M. Berwick

It was very late at night, and she was very, very sick. I was a brand new intern on my first rotation in the intensive care unit of one of the most revered hospitals in America. As the traditions of training had it in those days, I was in charge, and, John, the JAR (junior assistant resident) was my backup, *if* I needed him.

She was in diabetic ketoacidosis. It's bizarre, but 33 years later, I think I remember the numbers: pH 6.4, potassium 8.2, blood sugar 1200. She was in a coma—near death. Her EKG looked like the Himalayas in profile.

I walked from the room, faced the wall near the coffee-stained desk in the far corner of the nurses' station and quietly began to cry. And I can still feel John's arm come across my shoulder, the moment of pause, and then, "Let's sit here for a minute. You can do this."

John pulled a black progress note sheet from the rack of papers above us, drew a series of columns, and labeled each one at the top: "Airway," "Sugar," "Potassium," "Acid-Base," "Sodium,"…and so on. I added some. Slowly, we filled each column with a list—a plan. "And what," John asked, "shall we do about her pH?" Gradually, the balance of talking shifted, from John, who started it, to me, as I reasoned my way through the challenges the patient and I faced. And what was overwhelming dissolved into order. What was impossible dissolved into action. What had defeated me, I defeated—we defeated. She went home in two days.

Method is everything.

Now, health care is on crisis. It is in ketoacidosis—pH 6.0. If you doubt it, go study the amazing Web site resource of the Commonwealth Fund (http://www.cmwf.org), or, better, read today's newspaper. The symptoms are no secret, and the lab tests are clear. High cost, low value, and, from the

viewpoint of the workforce, not much fun. What are we to do?

Crying is an option. It always is. So is blaming—rather easy. But how about changing? How about learning? Could we do that instead?

This book, *Practice-Based Learning and Improvement: A Clinical Improvement Action Guide,* Second Edition, offers health professionals a path toward the positive change our health system requires. Here is a method that can guide well-intentioned, highly motivated, and deeply caring clinicians in the essential and ongoing work of quality improvement. Care for the patient, improve the patient's health; care for the system of care, improve the system's health.

The reader will find in these pages practical tools and techniques to stimulate both professional development and real-time optimization of clinical care, such as the following:

- Interventions that clarify local problems and identify striking improvement opportunities
- Worksheets that guide clinical improvements for populations in diverse practice settings
- Approaches to balanced measurement of care-related quality and costs
- Benchmarking methods that reveal "best of the best" practices yielding consistently superior results
- Innovations in professional education that build improvement know-how into the core curriculum for future clinicians
- Strategies implemented by pathbreaking health care organizations (such as Intermountain Health Care, the Vermont Oxford Network, the Dartmouth Spine Center) to design, measure, and transform clinical care systems

Given the will to do the best, *method is everything*. I don't know where John is today, but in helping me to organize my thinking, to approach that desperately ill woman's needs as a teachable, learnable system of causes, effects, and interactions, to help me see that my desperation was the signal of disorganization, not of impossibility, John made me into a doctor. He will never know how grateful I am. He linked progress to knowledge, success to learning, answers to questions.

Practice-based learning and improvement is the same thing. The patient is care itself. The disease is care as it should not be. The object of action is not a body, but a system of work. In this book, Eugene Nelson, Paul Batalden, and Joel Lazar offer to place their arms, as John once did to me, around the shoulders of the all too many professionals, staff, and leaders in health care today who wish they could help but don't know how, and who are crying, quietly. "Sit here," they say, "you can do this."

You can do this.

Method is everything.

Acknowledgments

Eugene C. Nelson,
Paul B. Batalden,
Joel S. Lazar

In an important sense, books are never done; they are just due. This may be especially true of a text on practice-based learning and improvement, whose central theme is the continually refined, but never completed work, of optimizing patient care.

We wish to offer special thanks to the large number of wonderful people whose generosity of time, spirit, and experience has made possible the creation and publication of the present book.

Our own work in practice-based learning and improvement has been stimulated by several thought and action leaders in this growing field. We have been inspired by the breakthrough achievements of David C. Leach, M.D., Executive Director, Accreditation Council for Graduate Medical Education, Chicago; David P. Stevens, M.D., Vice President, American Association of Medical Colleges, Washington, D.C.; Donald M. Berwick, M.D., M.P.H., President and Chief Executive Officer; Maureen Bisognano, Vice President and Chief Operating Officer; and Thomas W. Nolan, Ph.D, Senior Fellow, Institute for Healthcare Improvement, Cambridge, Massachusetts; Stephen Jencks, M.D., M.P.H., Director, Quality Improvement Group, Office of Clinical Standards and Quality, Centers for Medicare and Medicaid Services; Dennis S. O'Leary M.D., President, The Joint Commission, Oakbrook Terrace, Illinois; and Sir Brian Jarman, M.D., Emeritus Professor, Imperial College Faculty of Medicine, London. The intellectual and practical work of these remarkable individuals has enriched our own thinking immensely.

We are indebted as well to the committed frontline and health system leaders whose achievements are featured in this book's several case studies. These leaders include Thomas A. Colacchio, M.D., and William T. Mroz, M.B.A., RN, who

launched the Bowel Surgery Improvement Team and helped its members in an impressive series of clinical accomplishments; James Valiant, M.D., whose curiosity about outcomes measurement has substantially improved care for patients with carpal tunnel syndrome; Robert Lloyd., Ph.D., and Lindsey Martin, M.P.H., who have been developing and promoting IHI's Whole System Measures; James N. Weinstein, D.O., M.S., who founded the Dartmouth Spine Center, which is now led by William A. Abdu, M.D., M.S.; William H. Edwards, M.D., and Caryn S. McCoy, M.S.N., R.N., who have worked together for many years to optimize care for low–birth weight infants and their parents; Brent C. James, M.D. M.Stat., who has pioneered the integration of quality improvement and quality control systems at Intermountain Healthcare; and Bruce Hamory, M.D., and Karen McKinley, M.B.A. R.N., who have championed improvement in the Geisinger Health System. The work of these and other individuals underscores the importance of translating abstract improvement concepts into concrete actions.

We are of course grateful to our contributing authors, who also include Kenneth P. Brin, M.D., Tina C. Foster, M.D., M.P.H., Marjorie M. Godfrey, M.S., R.N., Julie K. Johnson, Ph.D., M.P.H., Christina C. Mahoney, M.S.N., R.N., M.S., Greg S. Ogrinc, M.D., M.S., Stephen K. Plume, M.D., and Jeanne Ryer, M.S. The contributors have graciously endured our deadlines and have continually rewarded us with their insights.

In addition, we are especially grateful to our editor, Steven Berman, and to the Executive Director of the Department of Publications, Catherine C. Hinckley, Ph.D., at Joint Commission Resources, for their support, encouragement, and advice throughout our journey of developing this book. We also appreciate the excellent professional writing skills that Jeanne Ryer, M.S, contributed to this book's predecessor, *Clinical Improvement Action Guide.*

Closer to home, we have been blessed with many colleagues at Dartmouth-Hitchcock Medical Center and Dartmouth Medical School who create unique conditions for the fostering of professional development and healthcare excellence. These colleagues also include Carl S. DeMatteo, M.D.; Elliott S. Fisher, M.D., M.P.H.; Nancy A. Formella, R.N., M.S.; Gerry T. O'Connor, Ph.D., D.Sc.; H. Worth Parker, M.D.; John E. Wennberg, M.D., M.P.H., John H. Wasson, M.D.; Louis A. Kazal, M.D.; Donald O. Kollisch, M.D, and Michael Zubkoff, Ph.D. Daniel F. Eubank, M.D., of the New Hampshire-Dartmouth Family Practice Residency has been an important mentor as well.

We also express our admiration for, and appreciation of, the following excellent administrative associates at Dartmouth: Linda L. Billings, Ph.D., who did extensive and yeoman work during manuscript preparation; and Joy McAvoy, Carol Johansen, and Gillian Jackson, who provided outstanding, unstinting, and ultra-reliable administrative and technical support.

We are humbly aware that none of the practice-based learning and improvement efforts described in this book could have been accomplished without thoughtful and generous feedback from our patients and their families. Clinical care is always a partnership, and the people whom we serve teach us continually how to serve them better. We have learned from our students as well, hundreds of them, whose insights challenge us repeatedly to refine our own methods and ideas. For this guidance and stimulation we are extremely grateful.

Finally, we extend our most heartfelt appreciation to our families: to Sandy, Alexis, Lucas, and Zach Nelson; to LaVonne, Maren, and Sonja Batalden; and to Barbara, Daniel, and Ben Lazar. We are conscious every day that our own work is sustained by their love and patience and support. It is only in this milieu that preparation of the current book could have been possible.

Start Close In*

By David Whyte

Start close in,
don't take the second step
or the third,
start with the first
thing
close in,
the step
you don't want to take.

Start with
the ground
you know,
the pale ground
beneath your feet,
your own
way of starting
the conversation.

Start with your own
question,
give up on other
people's questions,
don't let them
smother something
simple.

To find
another's voice,
follow
your own voice,

wait until
that voice
becomes a
private ear
listening
to another.

Start right now
take a small step
you can call your own
don't follow
someone else's
heroics, be humble
and focused,
start close in,
don't mistake
that other
for your own.

Start close in,
don't take
the second step
or the third,
start with the first
thing
close in,
the step
you don't want to take.

*Reprinted from Whyte D.: *River Flow: New & Selected Poems 1984–2007* by permission of the Many Rivers Press, Langley, Washington, 2007.

INTRODUCTION

Eugene C. Nelson,
Paul B. Batalden,
Joel S. Lazar

Start close in....
Start with
the ground
you know,
the pale ground
beneath your feet
—David Whyte, "Start Close In"[1]

The Ground We Know

Every clinician knows, as does every patient, every loved one, every participant in the process of care—every one of us knows that health care can be improved.

We know this, although, as clinicians, we likely received no formal training in improvement methods during our professional education, nor was the expectation of continuous quality improvement work built explicitly into our job descriptions. We know it as recipients of those same health services, although as patients we probably trust and respect our own providers, who are committed to the relief of our suffering and the promotion of our well-being.

We know it, ultimately, because we have experienced in our professional or personal lives the significant gap between what is possible in modern medicine and what in reality often transpires. Indeed, despite the talents and compassion and best intentions of all participants, we deliver, receive, or manage clinical service in systems that have not been designed for best care. Abundant data now support this assertion. In 1999, the Institute of Medicine (IOM) issued its report *To Err Is Human: Building a Safer Health System,* which documented nearly 100,000 needless health care system–related deaths in the United States per year.[2] More recent surveys indicate that Americans receive only 50% to 60% of recommended interventions for acute, chronic, and preventive care needs.[3] The IOM concluded in its 2001 *Crossing the Quality Chasm* report that significant deficiencies in the design of our current system consistently undermine delivery of the highest quality care.[4]

These IOM reports demand our attention at a time when other important health care developments create "tension for change"[5] as well. In recent years, for example, institutional and even individual practitioner measures of health care quality, safety, and cost have been made increasingly transparent to patients, payers, and the public. In 2003 and 2004, the National Quality Forum, a not-for-profit membership organization dedicated to developing and implementing a national strategy for health care quality measurement and reporting, called for public release of quality and safety measures by hospitals, nursing homes, and other health care providers.[6] Moreover, the Centers for Medicare & Medicaid Services (CMS) and The Joint Commission have mandated public reporting by hospitals of core quality measures pertinent to common health conditions and patient perceptions.[7]

In parallel with this transition to increased transparency, health care payment systems are moving in the direction of value-based purchasing to reward higher quality and lower costs. Private insurers and now Medicare have begun to base reimbursement for chronic disease management on providers' measurable compliance with evidence-based quality recommendations, and trends toward "value-based purchasing" of health services will certainly continue.[8] Metrics for both quality and cost will grow more accurate and pervasive, so that informed patients might selectively entrust their care and informed purchasers can selectively channel their beneficiaries to health care organizations that deliver highest value.

At the same time, the Accreditation Council for Graduate Medical Education (ACGME) has clarified and expanded the expected skill sets of physicians, and has mandated the explicit building of these skills into professional education. In 1999 ACGME officially endorsed six general competencies that all graduates of board-certified residency programs must master: patient care, medical knowledge, professionalism, systems-based practice, interpersonal and communication skills, and (notably) practice-based learning and improvement.[9] Undergraduate and graduate medical training programs are developing formal tracking systems to document achievement of these competency goals, and continuing education for practicing physicians will increasingly target these goals as well.

Thus, "the ground we know" is shifting. The imperative to achieve better clinical outcomes, to improve system performance, and to build improvement knowledge into professional training and development is increasingly apparent. This new work might challenge us and at times even threaten us, but it also invites us to rethink the way we do our work, so that we can do the work better.

It is precisely this invitation that informs our new book. The time has come to connect system improvement with both clinical practice and clinical learning. "Starting close in," [with] "the ground we know," we can add value to the care we offer our patients, and we can increase satisfaction in our own professional lives.

Our Daily Work

Two of us [E.C.N. and P.B.B.] recall a three-day course, "Quality 101," which we offered in 1988 to leaders of the Hospital Corporation of America (HCA). The setting was HCA's corporate headquarters in Nashville, Tennessee, and the subject matter was the introduction of modern improvement thinking into mainstream healthcare delivery. A nurse who had previously been silent raised her hand on the course's final day. She declared with excitement, "Dr. Batalden, I finally get it! We all have two jobs: to do our work and to improve our work!"

This nurse from Nashville did "get it," and her straightforward expression of our "two jobs" has remained in our minds ever since. The message is a simple and essential one, but too often it is overlooked in discussions of health care quality. Because (until very recently) practice-based learning and improvement has not been built explicitly into clinicians' professional training or recertification, and because improvement work is not routinely embraced as a regular responsibility of either clinicians or academicians, many practitioners assume that only special quality improvement committees are equipped and empowered to engage in such efforts. When individuals (or groups) are "assigned" to a specific improvement proj-

ect, the commitment of time and energy might thus feel like "extra work" (with all the negative associations of such labeling). Only infrequently is it recognized as "essential work."

We emphasize repeatedly in *Practice-Based Learning and Improvement: A Clinical Improvement Action Guide,* as the nurse from Nashville discovered in 1988, that all health care professionals do indeed have two jobs: to *do* the work, and to *improve* the work; we assert that these mutually supportive endeavors must be built into clinical and nonclinical services every day, in all parts of the system. What might such a health care system look like, if this "two job" message were universally adopted? We can imagine a culture of quality that engaged everyone in the improvement process. Staff would be recruited with this priority specifically in mind. The concept would be built into orientation, performance expectations, spontaneous coaching of staff by leaders, and periodic performance reviews. Managers at every level of the organization would ask their staff: "So what are you currently working on to make things better around here? What tests of change are you running? What do your data show? Does it make sense to try spreading this to other places?" Leaders would ensure that all staff members have the knowledge, skills and tools to build improvement into daily work.

Such places do exist in health care today, though they are uncommon. We have witnessed the effective development of improvement programs in diverse health systems around the world—in Cincinnati, at Cincinnati Children's Medical Center; in Seattle, at Virginia Mason Hospital and Medical Center; in Florence, South Carolina, at McLeod Regional Medical Center; in Bangor, Maine, at Evergreen Medical Practice; in Salt Lake City, at Intermountain Healthcare; in Pittsburgh, at Shadyside Hospital; in the Jönköping (Sweden) County Council Health System; in Stockholm, at the Karolinska Institute; and in several communities throughout the United Kingdom. An important goal for all health care leaders and practitioners is to generate similar success in larger numbers of local settings, so that the practice of quality improvement becomes normal activity in the daily work of clinicians.

The Purpose of this Book

We are motivated by precisely this vision of developing a culture of quality in health care systems, and we endeavor in *Practice-Based Learning and Improvement: A Clinical Improvement Action Guide* to empower health professionals to realize this vision in their own practices. We assume from the outset (and reiterate in the chapters ahead) that quality improvement is the work of everyone and that it must be directed simultaneously to the mutually supportive goals of better clinical outcomes, better system performance, and better professional training and development.

To support these goals, we offer both a conceptual framework and practical tools, and we combine the two in exercises and case studies that challenge the reader to identify local resources and opportunities, to define improvement tasks more precisely, and to *act*, "starting close in" as Whyte's poem reminds us, so that positive and meaningful change becomes synonymous with clinical work itself.

Because quality improvement is indeed the work of everyone, we have developed this book with several audiences in mind—clinicians, teachers and mentors of clinicians, participants of interdisciplinary work groups, and leaders of health care programs and systems. Clinicians will discover practical improvement tools that are designed for use in real-world settings of care. The Clinical Value Compass in particular will support practitioners' identification of worthy goals for improvement, clarification of target measures, analysis and benchmarking of current practice patterns, and design of specific tests of local change. Educators can adapt these same ideas and instruments for didactic purposes and can apply specific principles and methods to develop action-based training modules for undergraduate and postgraduate clinician learners. Interdisciplinary work groups will find similar support for their educational and improvement projects, with special attention to strategies and techniques that build upon the unique knowledge and skills of all participants. Health care leaders will recognize the applicability of value compass thinking in management settings, where it can stimulate structured planning and implementation of new initiatives and facilitate monitoring of balanced outcome measures in domains of patient care quality, health care costs, and system performance.

The Trajectory of Practice-Based Learning and Improvement

We invite readers to join us on a journey of both action and reflection. Although busy clinicians might choose to "sample" individual chapters that are relevant to specific concerns, we have constructed *Practice-Based Learning and Improvement: A Clinical Improvement Action Guide* with a developmental trajectory in mind. Beginning in Chapter 1 and proceeding in order, we move from the

general to the specific, and then, in Chapters 6 through 9, "circle back," after simpler concepts have been mastered, to higher-order syntheses with more general application. In this manner, we hope to track the natural progression of action-based learning, and we encourage readers to follow the same path. Clinicians who are new to the field might thus wish to dedicate more time to the basic principles of early chapters (1 through 5), while practitioners with greater quality improvement experience might proceed more quickly to the advanced discussion in the later chapters (6 through 9).

Chapter 1 introduces essential knowledge systems that support the work of practice-based learning and improvement. This conceptual framework establishes relevant context for the more task-oriented chapters that follow. Improvement work itself begins in Chapter 2, and with it the process of practice-based learning in local contexts of care. We lead the reader through a brainstorming exercise that generates multiple new ideas for improvement, building up resources available to all of us in our daily work. In Chapter 3 these ideas are refined and made operational. The Clinical Improvement Worksheet guides both individual practitioners and larger work groups in identifying and targeting specific aims and in developing specific tests of change that support measurable and sustainable improvement in both processes and outcomes of care.

The Clinical Value Compass, described in detail in Chapter 4, is a conceptual and practical centerpiece of practice-based learning and improvement, and indeed the "arrows" of this value compass point backward and forward to the other chapters of our text. We focus here on measuring what matters most: patient outcomes. But we define these outcomes in balanced terms that honor not only clinical or biological parameters but also measures of functional status, patient perception and satisfaction, and cost. Case studies demonstrate the Clinical Value Compass's utility in clarifying and measuring outcomes in all these important domains.

In Chapter 5 we turn attention outward from local contexts of care and introduce benchmarking techniques that facilitate scanning of the external environment for comparative practice patterns. The Clinical Benchmarking Worksheet can be used in concert with the Clinical Value Compass to answer the following important questions: Who is getting the best outcomes? What are they doing to get those best outcomes? What does the evidence base tell us about achieving outcomes of similar quality?

Subsequent chapters broaden and deepen the scope of both action and understanding in practice-based learning and improvement. Chapter 6 invites readers to explore change concepts that direct attention to high-leverage improvement opportunities. We consider ten core concepts that have proven especially valuable in our own work, and we demonstrate their applicability in an extended case study. Chapter 8 provides a different, development-focused perspective on these same themes. Two medical educators reflect on the evolving needs of clinician-learners as they mature into competent practitioners of improvement. If the achievement of better clinical outcomes and better systems performance is indeed the work of everyone, then how do we build developmentally appropriate experiences of practice-based learning and improvement into every stage of professional training, from undergraduate medical education, to postgraduate residency, to board recertification?

As health professionals achieve competency and even proficiency in the practice of clinical improvement, perspectives and possibilities will extend even further. Chapters 7 and 9 present advanced applications of practice-based learning and improvement, noting that even systemwide achievements in quality and outcome are built on simpler principles of change that we have already reviewed. Thus, in Chapter 7, an international leader of healthcare quality management describes Clinical Programs and Clinical Process Models (CPMs), the sophisticated and powerful approach that enables Intermountain Healthcare to build quality improvement and control into frontline microsystems of care. In this extended case study, we see that familiar change concepts and techniques inform a well-designed quality infrastructure, which in turn generates reliable and responsive patient-centered care, ongoing measurement of outcomes, and continuous improvement that relies upon and contributes to evolving biomedical knowledge.

Finally, in Chapter 9, we make the connections between local and systemwide change even more explicit, and we highlight progressively broader applications of practice-based learning and improvement. In a series of illustrative case studies, we recapitulate and extend the forms of knowledge and action that previous chapters have introduced, but we now find that local strategies and techniques of implementation are extended to regional, national, and even international levels.

To support the reader in adapting concepts and methods to settings of local relevance, we also include a series of Appendices that include specific tools that we have found valuable in our own work:

- *Appendix A* provides a full set of improvement worksheets for use by individual practitioners or larger improvement teams.
- *Appendix B* describes qualitative research methods and provides worksheets specifically adapted for qualitative learning and improvement.
- *Appendix C* offers validated patient report measures for evaluation of clinical, functional, satisfaction, and cost outcomes.
- *Appendix D* summarizes principles and practices of measurement in the process of clinical improvement.
- *Appendix E* lists several Web site resources that can further stimulate and support practice-based learning and improvement efforts.

In addition, a Glossary includes brief definitions for many terms used in our text that might be unfamiliar to some readers.

Starting Close In

We thus invite the reader to "start close in," to reflect on familiar patterns of practice, to acknowledge local barriers to the optimization of care, but also to recognize local resources (human and material) that can support and sustain improvement in this care. Those resources are in fact abundant. Our hope is that this book will be counted among them, and, more important, that it will stimulate readers to engage *all* resources in a new and more effective manner. The result, we believe, will be a new appreciation of the job of everyone, the simultaneous doing and improving of our work. Not only our patients, but also we ourselves, will benefit from this worthy effort.

References

1. Whyte D.: *"Start Close In."* In *River Flow: New & Selected Poems 1984–2007.* Langley, WA: Many Rivers Press, 2007.
2. Institute of Medicine: *To Err Is Human: Building a Safer Health System.* Washington, D.C.: National Academy Press, 1999.
3. McGlynn E., et al: The quality of health care delivered to adults in the United States. *N Engl J Med* 348:2635–2645, Jun. 26, 2003.
4. Institute of Medicine: *Crossing the Quality Chasm: A New Health System for the 21st Century.* Washington, DC: National Academy Press, 2001.
5. Gustafson D.H., Cats-Baril W.L., Alemi F.: *Systems to Support Health Policy Analysis: Theory, Models, and Uses.* Ann Arbor, MI.: Health Administration Press, 1992.
6. National Quality Forum: *Reports.* http://www.quality forum.org/publications/reports/ (accessed May 23, 2007).

7. The Joint Commission: *Performance Measurement Initiatives.* http://www.jointcommission.org/PerformanceMeasurement/ PerformanceMeasurement/ (accessed May 23, 2007).
8. Trude S., Au M., Christianson J.B.: Health plan pay-for-performance strategies. *Am J Manag Care* 12:537–542, Sep. 2006.
9. Accreditation Council for Graduate Medical Education (ACGME): *ACGME Outcome Project: Competencies.* http://www.acgme.org/outcome/comp/compHome.asp (accessed May 23, 2007).

Understanding Clinical Improvement: Foundations of Knowledge for Change in Health Care Systems

Eugene C. Nelson, Paul B. Batalden, Joel S. Lazar, Kenneth P. Brin

The dilemma of rigor or relevance may be resolved if we can develop an epistemology of practice which places technical problem solving within a broader context of reflective inquiry, shows how reflection-in-action may be rigorous in its own right, and links the art of practice in uncertainty and uniqueness to the scientist's art of research. —Donald A. Schön[1(p. 69)]

In the unique and ever-changing context of real world clinical practice, what forms of knowledge and skill are required to achieve the best patient care? Abundant data make clear that clinicians' technical competence and scientific knowledge, although necessary components of such care, are not sufficient to guarantee its consistent delivery. Numerous studies document the significant chasm between biomedical knowledge, which is extensive, and optimal clinical outcomes, which are frequently not achieved.[2,3] To close this gap, and to ensure care that is safe, effective, and open to continuous reflection and improvement, health professionals must connect their scientific knowledge to daily work patterns and embrace opportunities for practice-based learning as they continually arise.

This chapter introduces a framework for understanding clinical quality and practice-based learning and continuous improvement as these become manifest in real-world health care settings. We begin by sharing a tale of two patients whose disparate outcomes, in the context of similar events, underscore the high stakes of clinical improvement work. We explore the foundations of quality improvement in clinical practice, with attention to systems of knowledge that are required for optimization of patient care, and we emphasize the evolving nature of health outcomes that are the final measure of this care. Discussions of continuous quality improvement must be grounded in the reality of clinicians' daily work and directed to the priorities of individual patients; our goal in this first chapter is to introduce language and concepts that support this vital discussion.

A Tale of Two Patients: An Actual Case*

At the end of one recent and typically busy office session, cardiologist Dr. William Barr paused to reflect on two male patients seen in his clinic that morning. Jim Burke and Tony Lamont were both in their late 50s, and both had suffered acute myocardial infarctions (AMIs) six months earlier. At today's visits, Dr. Barr was impressed that despite the similarity of these patients' initial cardiac events, their clinical outcomes were dramatically different.

Jim Burke reported with satisfaction that he felt considerably healthier now than he had before his AMI. He had lost 20 pounds through a regimen of healthy diet and regular exercise and had experienced no recurrence of anginal symptoms. He had returned to his job and engaged in both work and play without functional limitation. His blood pressure and serum lipid levels were in optimal range, as specified by evidence-based guidelines. He felt, overall, quite free from anxiety, and expressed rational optimism regarding his future health outlook. He voiced pleasure with the cardiac care he had received, and bragged that he felt "better now than I have in years."

Tony Lamont, on the other hand, was decidedly unhappy with his current clinical status, and for good reason. He had been unable to return to prior work because of recurrent episodes of shortness of breath and palpitations; his energy and exertional tolerance were poor because of sustained

Names in this case and all cases in the book are fictitious.

myocardial damage. He had been hospitalized twice after experiencing his initial AMI and was concerned about the large medical expenses and significant co-payments that had depleted his savings. His cardiac risk profile remained suboptimal (hypercholesterolemia, hypertension, overweight, clinical anxiety); he acknowledged feeling "down in the dumps" and expressed genuine concern about his future. Tony had scheduled today's visit with Dr. Barr for a second opinion. Although he liked his own physician, he also hoped that a new perspective might help him to recover his sense of lost health and to get his life "back on track."

As Dr. Barr reflected on these divergent clinical outcomes and on the variation in clinical care which (his chart review suggested) was a likely contributor to this divergence, he grew aware of his own ambivalent response. Jim's successful recovery made clear what was possible in the provision of modern medical care, but Tony's unfortunate decline highlighted persistent barriers to delivery of that optimal care in his own community. Although differences in both premorbid health status and precise location of coronary obstruction will of course significantly affect

post-AMI outcomes, these differences did not appear substantial in the case of Jim and Tony. More significant were variations in the content, timing, and coordination of specific interventions. Details of both men's hospital and posthospital therapy are elaborated in Sidebar 1-1 (below).

What is most notable for our current discussion is Dr. Barr's appreciation that the clinical professionals involved in these two patients' care did not differ significantly in terms of scientific knowledge. Well-trained physicians and staff were employed at the sites where each man received their initial treatment. In one case, however, systemwide strategies had been established to ensure that scientific knowledge was appropriately implemented; in the other case, this same scientific knowledge was not coupled with work processes at the front line of care to support thorough and timely delivery of evidence-based interventions. The consequences of this difference will continue to be felt not only by Jim and Tony, but also by their families, their employers, and the payers of their increasingly divergent health care costs.

SIDEBAR 1-1. **A Tale of Two Patients, Continued**

As the main chapter text suggests, differences in premorbid health status and in the precise location of coronary obstruction were less substantial, in the cases of Jim and Tony, than were variations in the content, timing, and coordination of specific interventions. Jim received evidenced-based interventions (including aspirin and a beta-blocker) within minutes of electrocardiographic (ECG) demonstration of his acute infarction, and phone contact with an interventional cardiologist (to expedite cardiac catheterization) was initiated simultaneously. Tony's ECG interpretation was delayed, and in the absence of standard orders and protocols, so was the initiation of cardiac medications and specialist consultation.

Both men underwent cardiac catheterization (though this occurred more promptly in Jim's case) and both were noted to have significant obstruction of the left anterior descending coronary artery (which supplies the anterior wall of the heart and contributes substantially to left ventricular function). Both men's vessels were successfully stented (reperfused) in the catheterization lab, and the patients were trans-

ferred to their hospitals' cardiac care units for ongoing monitoring.

Subsequent to reperfusion, but still within the 24 hours of presentation, Jim was started on two additional medications, an angiotensin-converting enzyme inhibitor and a statin, to support cardiac pump function and to lower serum cholesterol. Tony received neither of these medications, though both were clinically indicated.

Within 48 hours of the presenting infarction, Jim received education from nursing staff and a hospital nutritionist, and both cardiac rehabilitation and timely follow-up appointments (with a primary care physician and with the outpatient cardiology clinic) were scheduled; specific appointment times were included with Jim's discharge instructions. Tony received some nursing education as well, though in a less thorough and coordinated manner. At discharge he was instructed to contact his primary care physician to arrange for a follow-up appointment. Several weeks later, at that follow-up visit, Tony reported ongoing exertional intolerance. No medications were added, but outpatient referral was made to a general cardiologist.

Foundations of Continuous Quality Improvement and Practice-Based Learning

If our goal is to improve the care of patients in real-world clinical settings and to achieve this improvement in the context of real world constraints on available resources, then we must commit ourselves to a process of reflection and learning that occurs in the "real time" of clinical practice itself. This process begins with an exploration of essential components in the work of quality improvement. Four foundational concepts require special attention: the priority of clinical outcomes, the necessity of universal engagement, the scope of improvement knowledge, and the functionality of clinical microsystems. The remainder of this chapter explores these four concepts in greater detail.

Clinical Outcomes Matter Most

In the final analysis, patients like Jim Burke and Tony Lamont are interested in clinicians' biomedical expertise and evidence-based care only insofar as they affect their clinical outcomes. As shall be elaborated, multiple forms of knowledge are required to create a system in which positive outcomes are most likely to occur. Before analyzing those forms of knowledge in greater detail, however, reflection on the outcomes themselves is in order. What domains of experience matter most to patients in real-world practice settings, and what outcomes should guide a clinical team's continuous efforts in performance improvement?

In the cases of Jim and Tony, the domains of relevant outcome are readily apparent. A first domain is essentially *biological:* the impact of AMI (and of its treatment) on cardiovascular morbidity and on mortality itself. What physiologic and pathophysiologic changes occur as a result of the coronary event, and what benefits and complications are associated with medical treatment? *Functional* health status is a second domain of great importance. After surviving their myocardial infarctions, can Jim and Tony return to their prior employment, can they participate actively, productively, and happily in community and family life, and can they reduce their risk of experiencing further cardiovascular problems? *Satisfaction against need* is another essential outcome domain. How do Jim and Tony themselves perceive the goodness of care and services they received, and to what extent have their needs and expectations for care been met? Finally, the fourth outcome domain of cost includes both direct medical expenses (incurred in the provision of clinical care) and indirect social costs that arise from lost

time at work, or from nonparticipation in other home-based or community-based affairs (that is, social role activities). Have these costs been minimized to the extent that is possible?

These four cardinal outcome domains are unified in the model of a Clinical Value Compass,[4,5] elaborated in greater detail in Chapter 4. Each outcome domain can be explored, measured, evaluated, and improved on using methods that are introduced later in this book. As depicted in Figure 1-1 (page 4), the Clinical Value Compass helps us to clarify favorable outcomes—in terms of biological and functional status, satisfaction, and cost— which Jim Burke now enjoys. This same value compass directs us to health service domains that could become targets of improvement in the care of Tony Lamont. "Value" can be understood as a ratio of improved clinical quality over costs, and the outcome-based emphasis of Jim's and Tony's Clinical Value Compasses permits us to assess these measures more precisely. Subsequent chapters of this book analyze components of value in much greater detail and explore means by which all clinicians can participate in sustaining and increasing value.

The Work of Everyone

Because practice-based learning and improvement are not routinely built into clinical training experiences nor explicitly mandated in most job descriptions, many health professionals consider such activities to be outside their usual scope of practice and responsibility. Quality improvement (QI) thus becomes synonymous with extra (rather than essential) work, an add-on to the practitioner's busy day. As a result, improvement tasks are delegated to special QI teams or resentfully squeezed in during administrative or personal time.

But when professionals can reflect on and reframe their implicit assumptions, clinical improvement is recognized as a necessary component of patient care itself. Highly effective practitioners and organizations, both inside and outside health care systems, understand that everyone has two jobs—to do the work and to improve the work. In health care (as in other service professions), this duality of activity, in turn, implies a third essential responsibility: Practitioners must endeavor *to learn* continually, so that both clinical care and its system-based improvement are performed with ever-increasing effectiveness and creativity.

Conceived in this way, the activities of patient care, practice improvement, and professional learning are interdependent and mutually supportive. As depicted in Figure

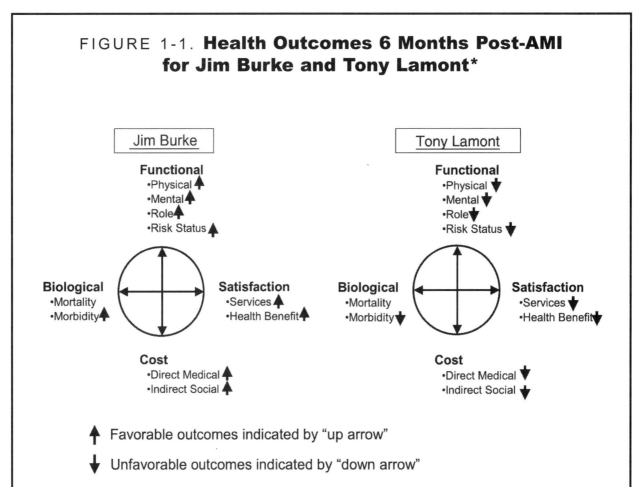

FIGURE 1-1. Health Outcomes 6 Months Post-AMI for Jim Burke and Tony Lamont*

Jim Burke

Functional
•Physical ▲
•Mental ▲
•Role ▲
•Risk Status ▲

Biological
•Mortality
•Morbidity ▲

Satisfaction
•Services ▲
•Health Benefit ▲

Cost
•Direct Medical ▲
•Indirect Social ▲

Tony Lamont

Functional
•Physical ▼
•Mental ▼
•Role ▼
•Risk Status ▼

Biological
•Mortality
•Morbidity ▼

Satisfaction
•Services ▼
•Health Benefit ▼

Cost
•Direct Medical ▼
•Indirect Social ▼

▲ Favorable outcomes indicated by "up arrow"

▼ Unfavorable outcomes indicated by "down arrow"

Figure 1-1. The Clinical Value Compass was used to clarify favorable outcomes for Jim Burke and health service domains that might become targets of improvement in the care of Tony Lamont—in terms of biological and functional status, satisfaction, and cost for both patients. *AMI, acute myocardial infarction.

1-2 (page 5), QI work is understood more inclusively as "the combined and unceasing efforts of everyone—health care professionals, patients and their families, researchers, payers, planners, educators—to make the changes that will lead to better patient outcomes (*health* in physical, psychological, and social domains), better system performance (*care* that is safe, timely, efficient, equitable, and so forth), and better professional development (*learning* new knowledge, skills, and values)."[6(p. 2)] Because these activities are indeed mutually supportive and universally assigned, there is no "extra" improvement work that is not really *essential* work, nor is there any time but now in which to perform it, nor anyone but ourselves (all of us) *who* can perform it.

Subsequent chapters return repeatedly to this assertion that better health outcomes, better care delivery, and better professional development are inextricably linked. There is optimism in this assertion, but also a challenge: The work of change and improvement must be under-

stood as an intrinsic part of everyone's job, every day, in all parts of the system. This is rewarding work, but it is by no means simple. We must therefore ask what new forms of knowledge and skill will be required. The remainder of this chapter specifically addresses this question.

The Clinical Improvement Equation

Experienced clinicians are well practiced in the art and skill of contextualizing scientific evidence—adapting general (and generic) recommendations to the unique needs, preferences, and capabilities of individual patients, and then monitoring the specific effects of this adaptation. "How does *that* clinical guideline apply to *this* patient in the office with me today?" We suggest that similar forms of translation and adaptation support continuous quality improvement at the level of health care systems, from local office settings to regional and even national networks of care. Here, too, both art and skill are required, and successful QI processes depend

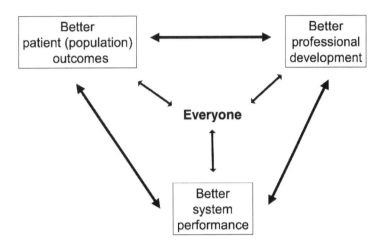

FIGURE 1-2. **Everyone Engaged: Better Patient Outcomes, Better System Performance, Better Professional Development**

Figure 1-2. Quality improvement work is understood to be the combined and unceasing efforts of everyone to make the changes that will lead to better patient outcomes, system performance, and professional development.

on very specific types of knowledge for their successful implementation.

Just as clinical practitioners combine knowledge of biomedical data with appreciation of individual patients' needs and preferences, so do practitioners of continuous quality improvement integrate knowledge of generalizable scientific evidence with unique clinical practice environments. We can reflect on this integration in a manner that supports our work in practice improvement. The following Clinical Improvement Equation[6] facilitates such reflective practice:

Generalizable Scientific Evidence + Particular Context →
Measured Performance Improvement

At first glance, this equation appears naively simplistic, but closer inspection reveals that it builds on complex and interdependent systems of knowledge. Indeed, not only the textual elements of this equation, but also its syntactic connectors, the "+" and "→" signs, embed specific operational tasks and depend on specific cognitive skills. Figure 1-3 (page 6) identifies the discrete tasks in more detail, whereas Figure 1-4 (page 7) illustrates essential forms of knowledge required for successful performance of each step. Let us probe the components of this Clinical Improvement Equation more deeply:

- **Generalizable Scientific Evidence.** The essential function here is *locating, acquiring, and evaluating biomedical knowledge.* Practitioners of clinical improvement must be skilled in forming answerable questions, retrieving and prioritizing information through Boolean searches, critically appraising retrieved studies, and interpreting the use of analytic techniques. Clinician-scientists navigate this system of knowledge with (relative) comfort, as it rehearses the familiar methodologies of academic medicine and engages the traditional information base of biomedical literature. By testing hypotheses in context-free settings, the methods of this analytic system build a necessary foundation. The resulting knowledge, however, resides in journals, books, and electronic databases, so it is far from sufficient to actualize improvement in real-world clinical settings.

- **Particular Context.** Practitioners of clinical improvement are adept at *characterizing unique practice environments,* and this skill depends on a knowledge system that receives far less attention in biomedical training and literature. Essential activities in this domain include interpreting data (both quantitative and qualitative) on local priorities and performance, assessing the populations' clinical and demographic characteristics, and evaluating the organizations' structures and interactions. What patterns, processes, and personalities support positive change, or hinder it, in this unique practice setting? What techniques might be applied to "diagnose" the local health system itself? In contrast to the first knowledge system—which eliminates consideration of local context by controlling for it in statistical models—this knowledge system focuses sharply on the particular setting and all that contributes to its "identity."

- **The "+" Sign.** The acquisition of both generalizable scientific evidence and particular context information does not itself ensure that these separate forms of knowledge shall be successfully integrated. An additional bridging domain of knowledge supports the *adapting of evidence and redesigning of practices.* Effective leaders of change know how to assess innovations for compatibility with the current system, how to design and sequence specific care algorithms to match locally available resources, and how to manage conflict and negotiation in the context of unique practice histories.

- **The "→" Sign.** When we bridge the general and the specific to identify strategies for local change that are grounded in scientific evidence, another domain of expertise is required to support the actual *execution of changes.* Champions of continuous quality improve-

ment are skilled in effective communication, in articulating a vision that compels group coherence, in supporting staff during stressful transitions, and in sustaining and embedding strategies for longer-term development. This knowledge system links strategic planning with human resource management to "make things really happen" in this particular place.

- **Measured Performance Improvement.** As described in subsequent chapters, successful improvement over time depends on reliable and recurrent *measurement of provider and system performance.* This method of measurement preserves time as a variable and seeks direct insight into the quality of results as these vary over time. Use of statistical process control charts, graphical displays, and other clinical assessment tools provides not only feedback data on improvement trends, but also "feed forward" information to facilitate point-of-care improvement in real-time practice.

Sustained and meaningful change is grounded in this full spectrum of knowledge systems derived from the Clinical Improvement Equation. The necessary skills can be learned (and we endeavor in this book to support that learning), and (more importantly) they can also be practiced! It is in this sense that continuous quality improvement and practice-based learning reveal their underlying identity. Our engagement in the work of improvement

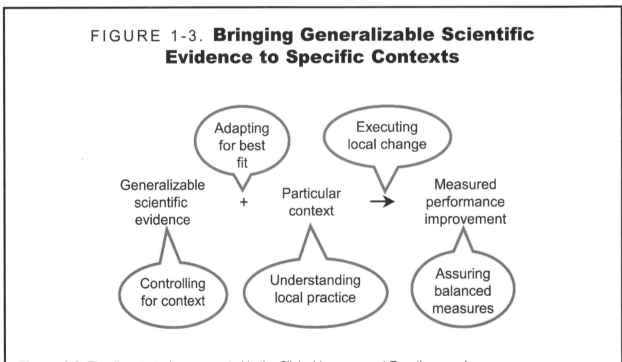

FIGURE 1-3. **Bringing Generalizable Scientific Evidence to Specific Contexts**

Figure 1-3. The discrete tasks represented in the Clinical Improvement Equation are shown.

FIGURE 1-4. **Knowledge Elements in the Science of Improvement**

Generalizable Scientific Evidence	**+**	**Particular Context**	**→**	**Measured Performance Improvement**
Locating, acquiring, and evaluating new knowledge	*Adapting evidence and redesigning practices*	*Characterizing practice environments*	*Executing changes*	*Measuring provider, system performance*
<u>Knowing how to:</u> • Define well-formulated, answerable questions • Identify/select good information sources, helpful reference librarians • Critically appraise retrieved studies & summaries of evidence	<u>Knowing how to:</u> • Formulate clear improvement aims • Identify alternative methods • Assess benefit/ compatibility • Select the best fit	<u>Knowing how to:</u> • Evaluate individual patients & patient groups • Assess current systems & processes • Understand successful changes in the context • Recognize local culture: what matters to people who work here	<u>Knowing how to:</u> • Identify & connect with what is strategically important for the future of the setting • Discern the ways things "work" and regularly get done locally • Attract and work interdependently with others in this setting • Recognize and honor good work • Foster the "unlearning" necessary to change	<u>Knowing how to:</u> • Design and interpret balanced measures of outcome • Use self-assessment • Measure and interpret performance over time, using statistical process control & graphic displays

Figure 1-4. The essential forms of knowledge required for successful performance of each step of the Clinical Improvement Equation are shown.

brings these separate knowledge systems to life and compels us to unify them for the ultimate purpose of optimizing patient care.

Systems and Microsystems of Care

Mastery of these multiple systems of knowledge is a daunting task for the individual practitioner. Fortunately, however, neither patient care nor quality improvement must be played as a "solo sport" in the twenty-first century. In both these clinical endeavors, the challenge and the opportunity to health care professionals are to sustain not only individual but collective competence and to support a cumulative "whole" of knowledge, skills, and experience that is greater than the sum of all persons' separate parts. Indeed, the efficacy of both clinical organizations and quality improvement teams derives in large part from the capacity of individuals to work together in, and *as*, well-integrated systems of care.

When Jim and Tony experienced their initial episodes of chest pain, they joined company in their respective

health care journeys not with isolated clinical practitioners but with sequential professional members of clinical teams, and indeed with members of multiple teams. The points of transition between members of each team and between the teams themselves were critical moments in the determination of overall quality of care. The speed of emergency room evaluation, the communication between clinical and nursing and administrative staff, the transport to the catheterization lab, the delivery of medication, the writing of coronary care unit admission orders, the discharge to home, the coordination of outpatient follow-up, the referral (or not) to cardiac rehabilitation services—each of these hand-off steps shifted performance responsibility to a new clinical team in Jim's and Tony's ongoing care.

There is great utility in identifying these smaller working groups as the true functional units of clinical care. We call such groups (of people, information, and technology) *clinical microsystems,* and elsewhere we have described their essential features in greater detail.[7,8] Microsystems are the small, naturally occurring frontline units that provide most clinical care to most people. These units can be characterized in terms of functional processes, patterns of communication, and the skill sets of each participant. They can also be understood organizationally, in relation to both the patients they serve and the larger health care systems of which they are a part.

As depicted in Figure 1-5 (below), microsystems can be conceptualized as one of several levels in an expanding series of health services and determinants. At the center of any health system is the individual or family with an active health need. Successive rings in the figure depict the patient in relationship with a clinician—whether a physician, nurse, or other trained provider—and then with the clinical microsystem itself, where patients, clinicians, and health care teams meet. Microsystems are supported in turn by larger mesosystems and macrosystems of care, which themselves are embedded in an economic, regulatory, and cultural environment that influences all levels of the health care system. These relationships are further characterized as follows:

- **Microsystems Are Both the "Ground" and the "Figure" of Patients' Experience in the Health Care System.** In their journeys from myocardial infarction to eventual wellness or illness, Jim and Tony moved through many different microsystems

of care. The emergency department, catheterization laboratory, cardiac care unit, cardiologist and generalist offices, and rehabilitation program were not only physical settings, the background against which health and illness were experienced, but were also active players, the "sharp end"[9(p. 10)] of the health care system where quality, and safety, satisfaction, and costs (that is, the Clinical Value Compass outcome domains) are continually created. Clinical outcomes depend on what patients such as Jim and Tony bring to each microsystem (for example, relevant information, prior health status, genetic endowment), and on what each microsystem does to (or with) that same patient (assessment, diagnosis, treatment, monitoring, and follow-up), as shown in Figure 1-6 (page 9).

- **Microsystems Are Linked, Tightly or Loosely, with Other Clinical Microsystems.** Collections of microsystems (for example, an emergency medical team squad, an emergency department, a catheterization lab, an inpatient unit for cardiac patients, a cardiology practice, a rehabilitation program) form mesosystems of care that serve patients with specific needs (for example, cardiac, obstetric, oncologic, or pediatric patients). Relationships within this greater

FIGURE 1-5. **The Relationship of Smaller and Larger Systems in Healthcare: Systems Embedded in Systems**

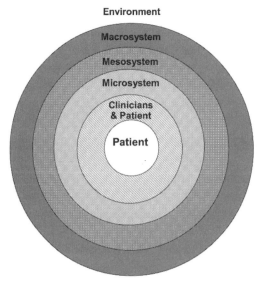

Figure 1-5. Microsystems can be conceptualized as one of several levels in an expanding series of health services and determinants.

mesosystem, as within the microsystem units themselves, might be implicit or explicit, and here again specific functional processes, patterns of communication, and participant competencies determine the overall quality of care that is provided.

- **Microsystems Are Often Embedded in Larger Macrosystems.** Frontline clinical units are often components of larger health systems (that is, macrosystems) that share common oversight and administrative infrastructure, such as hospitals, group practices, or networks of health care facilities. The microsystem relies on this larger macrosystem to provide clinical and administrative supports that are essential to both patient care and business operations. Such support might include diagnostic testing, medical records management, transportation, pharmacy, billing, and informatics coordination. The large health system, in turn, depends on clinical microsystems to deliver the "company product," that is, to provide the right care in the right way at the right time, so that patients receive maximum achievable benefit through the most efficient use of available resources.

Outcomes, Improvement, and Microsystems of Care

How do the Clinical Value Compass, the Clinical Improvement Equation, and high-performing clinical microsystems come together to optimize patient care in local contexts and to support the practice-based learning of health professionals? As suggested earlier, the final measures of quality are patient-oriented outcomes—not the "ideal" outcomes that inspire us in randomized, context-free, clinical trials (important as these are), but the

real-world outcomes that are achieved by clinical microsystems in particular health care settings, one patient at a time. The Clinical Value Compass brings clarity to a wide range of outcomes available for continuous improvement work, whereas the Clinical Improvement Equation maps specific skills and knowledge systems that a high-functioning microsystem must (collectively) master to meet those quality goals. Moreover, because microsystems are themselves composed not only of health care providers but also the evolving information, interactions, and technical resources that connect and support these providers, such functional units of care become both the context and the substrate for practice-based learning and professional development. These relationships are depicted in Figure 1-7 (page 10) and Figure 1-8 (page 10).

Jim's and Tony's divergent health trajectories highlight several further improvement-related outcome characteristics:

- **Health Outcomes Evolve Over Time.** Each step in the delivery of care contributes not only to immediate outcomes but also to the trajectory and priority of subsequent outcomes. Jim's and Tony's clinical needs changed over time (from "saving my life" to "saving the quality of my life"), and so too did their perceptions of services directed toward meeting those needs. Clinical care and system improvement are not static events but dynamic processes that require flexibility and creativity from all participants.

- **There Are Multiple Types of Health Care Outcomes.** Quality can and should be assessed in multiple outcome domains simultaneously, and these domains (as defined by the Clinical Value Compass) affect one another continually. Jim's satisfaction with

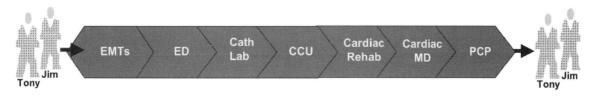

FIGURE 1-6. **The Clinical Microsystems that Cared for Two AMI Patients on Their Health Care Journeys***

Figure 1-6. The clinical microsystems that Jim Burke and Tony Lamont encountered are shown.
* AMI, acute myocardial infarction; EMTs, emergency medical technicians; ED, emergency department; Cath Lab, coronary catheterization laboratory; CCU, coronary care unit; Cardiac Rehab, cardiac rehabilitation; Cardiac MD, cardiologist practice; PCP, primary care physician practice.

FIGURE 1-7. **Clinical Microsystems, the Improvement Equation, and Value Compass Outcomes in the Flow of a Health Care Delivery System***

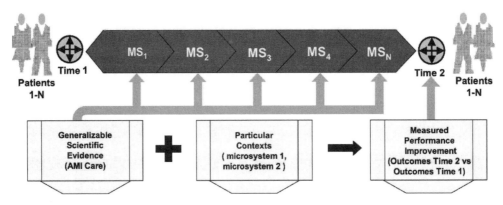

Figure 1-7. Microsystems, which are themselves composed not only of health care providers but also the evolving information, interactions, and technical resources that connect and support these providers, become both the context and the substrate for practice-based learning and professional development.
* AMI, acute myocardial infarction; MS, microsystem.

FIGURE 1-8. **Everyone Engaged in Relation to the Value Compass, Clinical Microsystems, and the Improvement Equation**

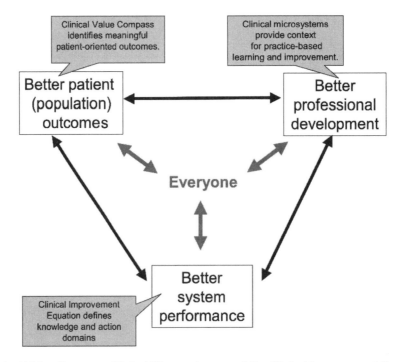

Figure 1-8. The Clinical Value Compass, Clinical Microsystems, and the Clinical Improvement Equation all play a role in contributing to better patient outcomes, system performance, and professional development.

care depended on his functional status (including his ability to resume employment); Tony's direct and indirect costs were related to optimization of biological markers of cardiac function. All these outcome domains are important and are likely to be prioritized differently at different times in the patient's health care journey. As previously emphasized, each outcome also suggests specific targets for future improvement work. The exercises in Chapter 2 build on the idea of multiple improvement targets and invite the clinical team to re-envision their improvement work in the broadest possible terms.

- **Outcome Measurement Is Essential for Quality Improvement.** The well-intentioned clinical professionals at Tony's hospital were unaccustomed to tracking process and outcome measures over time, and as a result they were simply unaware of their own suboptimal performance. As depicted in the Clinical Improvement Equation, the capacity to measure one's own performance is an essential competency in the science and practice of quality improvement. Subsequent chapters (especially Chapters 4 and 7) argue that active use of quantitative self-assessment greatly empowers clinical microsystems to improve their own work in real time. In this context, professional development and practice-based learning need not be burdensome "extra tasks" that are squeezed into a busy day. Instead, the self-monitoring of selected performance variables builds development and learning into clinical care itself.

Final Reflections on Clinical Improvement

Motivated by his separate encounters with Jim Burke and Tony Lamont, Dr. Barr continued his own process of reflection in the days and weeks ahead. He recognized in subsequent explorations the extent to which value compass thinking, improvement-oriented knowledge systems, and microsystem organization had been actively embraced by the hospital where Jim (but not Tony) had received his initial cardiac care.

Dr. Barr came to three further conclusions, which we offer here:

- **Successful Improvement Comes from Actualizing the Clinical Improvement Equation in Each and Every Clinical Encounter.** High-functioning microsystems develop protocols and pathways to manage routine interventions with great efficiency, but quality "happens" one patient at a time.

Consistent delivery of such quality requires both rigorous attention to the latest scientific evidence and specific adaptation to well-understood individual contexts. Available evidence, both general and contextual, must be integrated in real time, that is, during the swift daily flow of patient care, and in circumstances that are often ambiguous. The reflective clinician and the reflective clinical unit embrace these challenges as continuous learning opportunities.

- **Improvement Is Too Big a Job to Delegate.** Because quality, safety, and efficiency are determined continuously in each clinical encounter, the responsibility for maintaining quality belongs to every member of the health care organization. As we have previously asserted, the expectation in clinical settings must be that every participant has two jobs—to do the work and to improve the work. Such a mandate requires that all clinicians, nurses, and administrative personnel receive basic training in modern quality improvement methods, and that all staff be encouraged and expected to use these skills in daily work. Leaders of health care organizations must in turn develop a broad and deep improvement infrastructure (for example, frontline training, informatics, safety systems) to nurture the growth of this quality culture.

- **Quality Measurement and Transparency Will Profoundly Change the Work of Health Care Systems.** Increasingly, evidence-based metrics are monitored by employers, regulators, payers, and the public itself.[10,11] Cardiac care performance data, for example, are published for most hospitals in the United States.[12] Private insurers and now Medicare have begun to base reimbursement for chronic disease management on providers' measurable compliance with evidence-based quality recommendations, and trends toward "value-based purchasing" of health services will certainly continue.[13] As metrics for both quality and cost (the two components of "value") grow more accurate, pervasive, and transparent, informed patients will selectively entrust their care — and informed purchasers will selectively channel their beneficiaries—to health care organizations that achieve the highest levels of demonstrable quality.

Conclusion

Several decades have passed since sociologist Robert Lynd implored his academic audience to ask of their own scholarly endeavors, "Knowledge for What?"[14] Clinician-scientists of the twenty-first century must ask themselves this same question. What are we trying to achieve in our front-line care of patients and populations, and what forms of knowledge, practice, and continuous learning are necessary to accomplish this goal?

In this first chapter we have developed a descriptive framework, a scaffolding of knowledge systems, that directs our collective attention to the challenges and opportunities of quality improvement in real-world practice settings. The Clinical Value Compass facilitates our understanding of patient-oriented outcomes, whereas the Clinical Improvement Equation reminds us that achievement of these outcomes depends on thoughtful adaptation of scientific evidence in locally defined contexts. This process of adaptation and implementation is the daily work of frontline clinical microsystems, which serve as both the supportive context and the substrate for practice-based learning and professional development. Success depends on both individual and collective competence in multiple domains of knowledge and skill.

Because several of these domains fall outside the usual training of clinicians, nurses, and health administrators, we are all on the steep slope of our learning curve. This is an exciting place to be, so long as we embrace our roles as continuous learners. In the chapters that follow, we begin our climb up this learning curve. Through specific exercises and case studies, we bring clinical improvement and practice-based learning into the daily work of patient care, with the goal of optimizing that care continuously in our own practice settings.

References

1. Schön D.A.: *The Reflective Practitioner: How Professionals Think in Action.* New York City: Basic Books, 1983.
2. Institute of Medicine: *Crossing the Quality Chasm: A New Health System for the 21st Century.* Washington, DC: National Academy Press, 2001.
3. Institute of Medicine: *To Err Is Human: Building a Safer Health System.* Washington, DC: National Academy Press, 2000.
4. Nelson E.C., et al.: Improving health care, Part 2: A clinical improvement worksheet and users' manual. *Jt Comm J Qual Improv* 22:531–548, Aug. 1996.
5. Nelson E.C., et al.: Improving health care, Part 1: The Clinical Value Compass. *Jt Comm J Qual Improv* 22:243–258, Apr. 1996.
6. Batalden P., Davidoff F.: What is "quality improvement" and how can it transform healthcare? *Qual Saf Health Care* 16:2–3, Feb. 2007.
7. Batalden P.B., et al.: Microsystems in health care: Part 9. Developing small clinical units to attain peak performance. *Jt Comm J Qual Saf* 29:575–585, Nov. 2003.
8. Nelson E.C., et al.: Microsystems in health care: Part 1. Learning from high-performing front-line clinical units. *Jt Comm J Qual Improv* 28:472–493, Sep. 2002.
9. Reason J.: *Managing the Risks of Organization Accidents.* Brookfield, VT: Ashgate, 1997.
10. Institute of Medicine: *Performance Measurement: Accelerating Improvement.* Washington, DC: National Academy Press, 2006.
11. National Quality Forum: *National Priorities for Healthcare Quality Measurement and Reporting.* Washington, DC: National Quality Forum, 2004.
12. National Quality Forum: *National Voluntary Consensus Standards for Hospital Care: An Initial Performance Measurement Set.* Washington, DC. National Quality Forum, 2003.
13. Porter M., Teisberg E.: *Redefining Health Care: Creating Value-Based Competition on Results.* Boston: Harvard Business School Publishing, 2006.
14. Lynd R.: *Knowledge for What: The Place of Social Science in American Culture.* Princeton, N.J.: Princeton University Press, 1939.

Initiating Change: Strategies to Target Clinical Care and Costs

Eugene C. Nelson, Paul B. Batalden, Jeanne C. Ryer

Quality is never an accident. Quality is always the result of intelligent effort. It begins with the intent to make a superior thing.
—John Ruskin[1]

Most health professionals understand that clinical systems, large and small, are in need of improvement, and that such improvement usually begins at the front line of patient care. But knowing how to initiate this improvement in local practice settings might be less intuitive. Certain barriers predictably impede the pursuit of positive change, not the least of which is the challenge to identify targets for change that are both meaningful and achievable. In this chapter we explore this challenge to the initiation of change in clinical settings and then pursue an extended exercise that generates multiple practice-based improvement ideas. We expect that this exercise will be tailored to the specific needs and constraints of individual clinical settings, but we believe that its general framework has broad applicability across practice types.

The Challenge(s) of Getting Started

We define practice-based learning and improvement as the reflective and iterative integration of observation and action, during clinical care, to enhance the knowledge and high-quality delivery of that care in every encounter. This is a laudable goal for all clinicians, and our patients expect nothing less from us. But initiation of such learning and improvement requires that we overcome significant obstacles to change in real-world settings. These obstacles can be personal, professional, or institutional, although resistance more commonly occurs at all three levels. Although change is, paradoxically, the one "constant" of our daily lives, it is also a potential threat to both individuals and organizations. Insofar as we conceptualize transitions and imperfections as problems to be avoided rather than challenges

to be embraced, we might find tenuous comfort in our retreat to the status quo.

Support from an organization's top leaders is vital to nurture and to sustain practice-based learning and improvement efforts over time, but some degree of improvement work is possible even in organizational cultures that lack systemwide support. Whatever our position and level of responsibility, each of us can create a climate of learning and improvement in our workplace that makes positive change not only possible but also regularly achievable.

An ancient Chinese proverb reminds us that the journey of a thousand miles begins with a single step. As we take our first step on the path to practice-based learning and clinical improvement, recognition of the following common challenges will simplify and support this journey.

Challenge 1. The Will to Be the Best

Ruskin observes, in the quotation that begins this chapter, that quality begins with "the intent to make a superior thing," the desire to find a better way—all the time, no matter what. The commitment to learn for the purpose of enhancing quality is an orientation to life and work, a conviction that the status quo is never good enough. This commitment balances *doing* what needs to be done (now) with reflecting on and *improving* what is done (now), so that the future will be better. The first challenge to overcome is resistance to this commitment itself.

We have found that honest reflection on our own work is often the most effective stimulus for embracing positive commitment to change. "Starting close in," as suggested in the

Introduction to this volume, we recognize the extent to which even small workplace inefficiencies can have large impacts on the care we deliver to our patients and on the satisfaction we derive from providing that care. Further reflection reveals that the converse is equally true: our past efforts to take the extra step, to attend with extra zeal and systematic rigor to specific patient needs, have greatly (even if slowly, one patient at a time) enhanced the quality of the care we provide, and of the care-giving experience itself. Sustainable practice-based learning and clinical improvement is all about "making a superior thing," internalizing this orientation to quality, so that we strive to achieve it every day.

Challenge 2. Time

Everyone is busy, and the best people for the job are often the busiest. But we all have the same amount of time in our day; we just choose to segment it differently on the basis of our personal and professional values. When we claim to lack time for improvement, we might in fact be expressing our tacit belief that improvement is not part of our regular work. By honoring the essential identity of "work" and "work improvement" and recognizing the efficiency that emerges from ongoing quality innovation, the busy and effective professional *builds* regular improvement time into work routines themselves. This can be achieved, for example, by holding daily team huddles (of brief dura-

tion) during which clinical operations are discussed and small tests of rapid change are planned. In this manner, frontline operations and continuous improvements become increasingly indistinguishable. In Sidebar 2-1 (below), we offer further recommendations that busy practitioners have found to be especially beneficial.

Concerns about time limitation and work efficiency have spawned a large time-management industry. Many people find books, tapes, seminars, and special tools on the topic to be helpful, and readers of the current chapter might wish to explore these resources. We support such efforts but advise individuals to be wary of a common trap: more time might be spent managing a complicated calendar system than is freed for doing what is really important.

In addition, many people mistake activity for accomplishment. Being busy does not guarantee productivity, and indeed it sometimes undermines our productivity. Valuable time can often be created for improvement projects by *eliminating* busywork or unnecessary activity. Later in this chapter we discuss the concept of *muda,* identifying common time-wasters whose elimination might enhance both productivity and quality.

Challenge 3. Know-How

Internal commitment and dedicated time are basic requirements for any improvement process, but specific know-

---

SIDEBAR 2-1. **Simple Time Management Techniques**

The real value of time management techniques is their ability to make visible our current choices and practices, thus exposing opportunities that were previously unseen. We all have exactly the same amount of time in each day: no variation here, except in how we use it. A number of simple strategies can help us to make the most of those 1,440 minutes:

- **Track the use of time.** Memory is not a good monitor; keep a careful time log for one or two weeks. This record will reveal multiple opportunities for increased efficiency.
- **Respect time, both personal and professional.** Be punctual. Prepare for meetings and phone calls, and keep on topic.
- **Manage meetings and mail.** Use huddles and focused meetings for greater productivity. Always start and end meetings on time. Stick

with the agenda, and keep minutes for later review. Manage mail (including e-mail) rapidly and ruthlessly.

- **Focus on what's important.** Remember the Pareto principle—80% of unfocused effort generates only 20% of results, and 80% of results come from only 20% of effort. Apply the Pareto principle to both personal and professional time.
- **Get on with it.** Unpleasant (but necessary) tasks are often the most time-consuming, precisely because we waste extra time in our avoidance of them. When confronted with such a task, just do it. As the old saying goes, "saw the big logs first." Procrastination and complex work-arounds almost always generate more undesirable work (and loss of time) in the future.

how is important as well. In the chapters that follow, we support the development of this know-how through detailed elaboration of practice-based clinical improvement strategies. But mastery of the entire canon of quality improvement (QI) techniques is not required to get started. Some general skills can be easily learned and applied creatively in both personal and professional domains.

We advise students of quality innovation to develop *personal* improvement projects early in their own process of practice-based learning. This experience enables individuals to "see" with different eyes, to appreciate that anything can be improved if we direct our attention toward it. In addition, many of the principles and methods employed in clinical improvement work are similarly applicable in personal contexts, and recognition of this overlap might serve as a valuable bridge to mastery with more formal methods.

Thus, in a master's degree course that one of us [P.B.B.] leads on improvement of health care delivery, students identify a personal goal, such as regular exercise, daily musical practice, or keeping up with e-mail correspondence. This goal becomes the focus of an improvement initiative for which implementation includes defining specific targets, anticipating potential barriers, developing detailed plans, recording observations on progress toward goals, and reflecting on outcomes. This extended exercise, based on a model developed by Roberts and Sergesketter[2] in a classic book, *Quality is Personal: A Foundation for Total Quality Management,* reveals to students the extent to which challenges to continuous improvement (clinical or otherwise) can be anticipated and overcome.

Too often, QI techniques are presented as a set of statistical and group process tools that will magically create improvement by themselves. When this doesn't happen, the tools might be prematurely dismissed as ineffective, and the motivation for improvement dismissed as ill conceived. The matching of personally and professionally meaningful improvement targets with well-chosen (but also flexibly applied) methods will increase the likelihood of success. Sidebar 2-2 (below) reviews some basic but very useful improvement resources.

SIDEBAR 2-2. **Useful Books for Improvement Projects**

Harry V. Roberts and Bernard F. Sergesketter's wonderful little book, *Quality Is Personal: A Foundation for Total Quality Management,* applies principles of quality management in personal settings.[1] Consider trying their ideas to enhance productivity and to learn improvement principles in contexts that are personally meaningful.

On the professional side, *The Improvement Guide: A Practical Approach to Enhancing Organizational Performance*[2] is a useful publication on making things work better in real-world businesses. The authors—Gerald Langley, Kevin Nolan, Thomas Nolan, Clifford Norman, and Lloyd Provost—explore change concepts and improvement principles that can be directly applied in clinical settings.

Additional helpful guide books are *The Memory Jogger II*[3] and *The Team Memory Jogger,*[4] the *Pocket Guide to Using Performance Improvement Tools,*[5] *The Power of Health Care Teams: Strategies for Success* by Kathleen Phillips,[6] *The Lean Six Sigma Pocket Toolbook,*[7] and *The Team Handbook,* 3rd edition[8]—all are packed with helpful techniques for managing group dynamics, supporting effective teamwork, improving work-flow processes, and solving practical problems.

References

1. Roberts H.V., Sergesketter B.F.: *Quality is Personal: A Foundation for Total Quality Management.* New York City: Free Press, 1993.
2. Langley G.J., et al.: *The Improvement Guide: A Practical Approach to Enhancing Organizational Performance.* San Francisco: Jossey-Bass Publishers, 1996.
3. Brassard M., Ritter D.: *The Memory Jogger II.* Methuen, MA: GOAL/QPC, 1994.
4. Brassard M., et al.: *The Team Memory Jogger.* Methuen, MA: GOAL/QPC, 1995.
5. Joint Commission on Accreditation of Healthcare Organizations: *Pocket Guide to Using Performance Improvement Tools.* Oakbrook Terrace, IL: Joint Commission, 1996.
6. Phillips K.: *The Power of Health Care Teams: Strategies for Success.* Oakbrook Terrace, IL: Joint Commission on Accreditation of Healthcare Organizations, 1997.
7. George M., et al.: *The Lean Six Sigma Pocket Toolbook.* New York City: McGraw Hill, 2005.
8. Scholtes P.R., Joiner B.L., Streibel B.J.: *The Team Handbook: How to Use Teams to Improve Quality,* 3rd ed. Madison, WI: Oriel Incorporated, 2003.

Challenge 4. Where to Start

Having overcome the prior challenges, many earnest practitioners remain unsure how to identify targets for clinical improvement itself. Individuals and teams are committed to quality and are knowledgeable of improvement principles and techniques but are unsure *where* to focus their energy and resources. A common next question is, "How do we find things to improve?" In the remainder of this chapter, we pursue a series of simple probes to identify multiple improvement opportunities available in every clinical practice.

Identifying Targets for Improvement in Clinical Care

As introduced in Chapter 1, the mutually supportive goals of clinical improvement work are better patient outcomes and better system performance. These goals, in turn, both support and are supported by better professional development. This is the work of everyone, which means that opportunities for improvement exist everywhere, in every facet of clinical care.

For individual practitioners who have difficulty getting started and for organized clinical teams that feel similarly stuck, the 14 action probes that follow will generate multiple improvement ideas to direct ongoing activity. For professionals already committed to specific quality concerns, this same exercise can focus improvement efforts, or can broaden the scope of contexts in which specific strategies are applied.

1. Talk to Insiders—Ask the Staff

Most clinical practices cannot afford the luxury of an external consulting group to identify potential improvement areas, but in fact, all health care settings are rich with internal experts: clinicians, nurses, receptionists, administrators, and many other participants who live the problems of service delivery every day. Indeed, staff members are among the best-informed consultants.

To get the benefit of their considerable expertise, ask any *five* people in the groups listed below to complete the following *two* statements:
1. The clinical work that needs to be improved if we want better patient outcomes is _____ (fill in the blank).
2. The reason(s) the system's performance is not as good as it could be is (are) _____ (fill in the blank).

Here is a list of staff to approach:
- New employees
- Employees who are getting ready to work elsewhere
- Receptionists
- House staff
- Volunteer workers
- Information desk staff
- Pharmacists
- Physicians
- Nurses
- Risk management staff
- Utilization review staff
- Billing office staff

2. Engage the Beneficiaries of Clinical Care—Ask Patients, Their Families, and Other Stakeholders

These direct and indirect beneficiaries of health care service have strong feelings about the quality of care we provide. Patients, their families, their employers, and their insurers will all be glad that we invited them into the discussion.

Ask any *five* people in the groups listed below to complete just *two* statements about the health care they receive:
1. The services this practice could improve to lessen my burden of illness include _____ (fill in the blank).
2. The things that I hear people complaining about in this practice include _____ (fill in the blank).

Address these questions to individuals on the following list:
- Patients
- Family members
- Employers
- Purchasers

3. See What Others Have Done—Explore the Literature

A growing number of public resources can facilitate identification of evidence-based guidelines and practice-based "best practices" for high-quality clinical care.

Look for improvement ideas in the following clinical guidelines and protocols:
- National Guideline Clearinghouse—a joint effort of the Agency for Healthcare Research and Quality (AHRQ), the American Association of Health Plans,

Use this workbook area for Sections 1 and 2.

The questions we asked were:

_____

_____

The groups we asked were:

_____

_____

And the answers were:

_____

_____

_____

_____

_____

_____

_____

_____

_____

Tapping into the experiences of staff members and stakeholders will generate many new improvement ideas.

and the American Medical Association—which provides full text and abstracts of clinical practice. (For more information on the National Guideline Clearinghouse, visit www.guideline.gov).

- Institute for Clinical Systems Improvement Web site: *Guidelines & More* (http://www.icsi.org/guidelines_ and_more/)[3]
- Care Process Models, Intermountain Healthcare (www.intermountainhealthcare.org/xp/public/ physician/clinicalprograms)

Specialist providers will be familiar with other guideline and protocol resources pertinent to particular clinical conditions.

4. Read About What Works—Check Out Case Study Reports

Challenges present in one practice setting have likely been confronted elsewhere as well. What targets have been identified, and what improvements achieved, in comparable practice settings?

Review illustrative case studies from journals and books, as well as Web sites of organizations that promote the quality and safety of health care. (We elaborate benchmarking techniques more fully in Chapter 5.)

5. Look at What Others Know about Local Practice—From the Outside Looking In

Transparency of performance is increasingly normative in health care systems.[4] Much of our clinical work is now monitored, quantified, and compared to external standards. (See Chapters 4 and 5 for further discussion.) Practitioners can gain valuable insight from data that has been externally collected on their own health care practices.

Review comparative results obtained from the following sources:

- Joint Commission survey results and performance data
- *Dartmouth Atlas of Healthcare* (www.dartmouthatlas.org[5])
- National Committee for Quality Assurance surveys and Health Plan Employer Data and Information Set results
- Quality Improvement Organization (QIO) studies
- Statewide databases on charges, costs, utilization, and outcomes

6. Treasure the Defects—If It's Broken, Fix It

Defect is a manufacturing term not fully integrated into health care workers' vocabularies, though in fact the phenomenon itself is very common in health care settings. Defects are mistakes, miscommunications, and errors of omission or commission that potentially jeopardize clinical care. In the majority of cases, these events are not the fault of a single person, but represent *symptoms* of a systemic process in need of improvement. If our goal is to reduce the frequency and negative impact of such events, we must paradoxically treasure them—that is, we must recognize them, measure them, and learn from them.

These manifestations of defects will show areas in need of improvement:

- Risk-management claims made (and paid)
- Complaints made by patients and families
- Medical error reports
- Adverse event reports
- Incident reports
- Quality assurance department reports
- Internal audit reports

7. Understand "Competitors"

Unless located in an unusual market area, most practices and clinical service programs "compete" in some manner to attract and to retain patients who are free to seek care in multiple settings. Improvement teams can learn from competitors who have attracted these patients by providing greater value in specific contexts. We advise teams to consider any clinical service in which they are not the region's low-cost, high-quality alternative, and to evaluate why the competitor is doing better.

Here is a list of potential sources of comparative cost and quality information:

- Local health maintenance organizations
- Statewide databases
- Employers and insurers
- Medicare databases

Use this workbook area for Sections 3, 4, and 5.

The outside sources we explored were:

_____

_____

_____

And the sources told us:

_____

_____

_____

Consulting these sources should produce many more improvement ideas.

8. Check Out the Customer Survey Results

Every organization performs surveys, and the resulting data can stimulate multiple improvement ideas.

Review surveys completed by the following groups:
- Patients and families
- Employees
- Medical staff
- Community residents
- Referring physicians

9. Understand the Current Process

Clinical processes connect team members to patients and to each other, and they are rich with opportunities for improvement. Identify and map the current ("as is") process of care (from both staff and patient perspectives), follow pathways of information flow, observe clinical steps, talk to people (patients, providers, support staff) about how things really work at the front line, and search for recurrent problems. One or more of the following process challenges might be an important target for improvement work:

- Bottlenecks, waits, delays, queuing, and interruptions
- Communication failures
- Errors and things going wrong
- Misplaced charts, equipment, or other necessary tools
- Steps that require exceptional effort to be performed properly
- Steps that involve multiple decisions
- Frustrations, irritations, and anger
- Rework and "do-overs"

10. Walk in Their Shoes—Play the Role

Most health care workers recall their own frustrations as a *recipient* of health care services. Participant observation can identify numerous steps in the clinical encounter that patients might experience as frustrating, and these are obvious targets for ongoing improvement.

Play the role of patient, or of another professional, and walk through the following steps:
- Being admitted
- Visiting a doctor
- Calling the doctor's office

Use this workbook area for Sections 6, 7, and 8.

Our standout defects are:

_____

_____

_____

Our noncompetitive service areas are:

_____

_____

_____

Our customer satisfaction surveys tell us we'd better look at:

_____

_____

_____

By tapping into the sources outlined in Sections 6, 7, and 8, several further improvement ideas can be generated.

Use this workbook area for Sections 9 and 10.

The internal systems we reviewed were:

_____

_____

_____

And the results pointed us to:

_____

_____

_____

Immersion in the care process will expose another set of target areas for improvement.

- Using an outpatient service
- Going to the emergency department

11. Review Internal Data

Health care organizations generate mountains of data. Using internal quantitative reports, identify the practice's or clinical program's top ten conditions in terms of any (or all) of the following parameters:
- Volume
- Costs
- Charges
- Amount of time spent
- Risk to patient
- Achievable Benefit Not Achieved ("ABNA," that is, the gap between what is possible and what is currently happening)

12. Identify Sink Holes of Temporary Help

Although periodic shifts in work flow might necessitate occasional hiring of temporary help (including float staff), the regular use of such workers can be cost inefficient and labor intensive (for staff who must oversee training), and might increase the risk of clinical or administrative errors.

Find the locations where temporary workers are hired most frequently. Redesign work to avoid the need for temps, or standardize work so that these temps produce error-free work.

13. Eliminate Waste—Look for Muda

Muda is a Japanese term that reflects the concept of shame arising from waste—wasted time, wasted effort, and wasted resources. (See Sidebar 2-3, page 22, for more details on *muda*.)

To find waste and to eliminate it, ask the same *five* people who served as insider problem-spotters (action probe 1, page 16) to complete the following *two* statements:
1. There's one thing we do all the time that accomplishes very little, and that's _____ (fill in the blank).
2. In my area, we always have plenty of _____, because only _____ ever uses them (fill in the blanks).

Ask the same *five* stakeholder groups identified earlier (action probe 2, page 16) to complete the following *two* statements:
1. At _____ (your institution), we always have to wait for_____ (fill in the blanks).
2. At _____ (your institution), we get _____, when what we really need is _____ (fill in the blanks).

Use this workbook area for Sections 11 and 12.

The top ten conditions in our system where improvement can have the biggest impact are:

_____

_____

_____

_____

_____

We must use our temporary help most often for:

_____

_____

_____

Analyzing internal systems has identified many more target areas for improvement.

Use this workbook area for Section 13.

We looked for *muda* in:

_____

_____

_____

_____

We found *muda* in:

_____

_____

_____

Waste is a frequent drain on organizations' resources. Exposing this waste generates several new improvement ideas to combat it.

SIDEBAR 2-3. **What's *Muda*?**

The Japanese word *muda* translates, roughly, to the concept of "futility and uselessness." Taichi Ohno, who led Toyota Motor Company's quality efforts for many years, used the term to signify activity without value, and in this sense *muda* can be found almost anywhere in our personal lives and organizational work. Indeed, as discussed below, we can recognize *muda* in several different forms. Our interpretation here is built on insights from Ohno, Roberts, Sergesketter, and others.

Muda **of resource consumption** is the use of work and supplies that consume time or money without adding value. If we imagine a meter to be running as each clinical process unfolds, we can identify parts of the process that consume resources without adding value. Muda is present when we admit patients the day before treatment, or when we ask these patients repeatedly for the same identifying and demographic information. In administrative work, we experience muda when starting meetings late, or when staying in these meetings though our presence is not required.

Muda **of inventory** is buildup of inventories (of services or products) that no one wants. In health care, this buildup is manifest in standing laboratory orders, in unused hospital beds, and in extensive menus of surgical supplies, staples, and suture materials.

Muda of action is the presence of unnecessary process steps. In health care, muda of action

(that is, action without the need for action) can be found in excessive testing, in convoluted scheduling rules, in reports that no one uses, and in continuous monitoring.

Muda **of transport** is the movement of employees, patients, equipment, or information without purpose. Examples in health care are easy to identify: movement of patients from labor to delivery to recovery rooms, uncoordinated transports to x-ray, changes of room because necessary equipment is unavailable, and multiple trips to the supply cart.

Muda **of waiting** occurs downstream when people or processes upstream are late. Again, examples are common in health care settings: Surgery is delayed because lab reports are unavailable, physicians or nurses must wait while information is updated in the computer, billing claims are delayed due to administrative barriers.

Muda **in meeting stakeholder needs** includes services or products that don't match priorities of patients or other beneficiaries. Patients are quite familiar with education materials that fail to answer their practical questions, with medications that don't get taken, and with hearing aids that stay in drawers. We also find muda of stakeholder needs in clinical pathways that never change and in pain management strategies that delay ambulation and discharge.

---

14. Probe the Process More Deeply—Use Change Concepts

As we discuss in greater detail in Chapter 6, change concepts are general high-leverage ideas that stimulate creative problem solving and promote novel ways of thinking—including generation of specific improvement strategies.[6,7]

Identify an important clinical service and apply one of these 10 change concepts (further elaborated in Chapter 6):

1. Modify input.
2. Combine steps.
3. Eliminate failures at handoffs between steps.
4. Eliminate a step.
5. Reorder the sequence of steps.
6. Change an element in the process by creating an arrangement with another party (that is, with a customer, supplier, or other individual who can perform the required step more effectively).
7. Replace a step with a better alternative.
8. Redesign production on the basis of knowledge of the service or product that is produced.
9. Redesign the service or product on the basis of knowledge of use of the service or product.
10. Redesign the process with knowledge of need and aim.

Use this workbook area for Section 14.

We chose the following clinical services:

_____

_____

We applied the change concept:

_____

_____

As a result, we are going to focus on:

_____

_____

By thinking about change concepts in local clinical systems, further improvement targets have been identified.

Narrowing the List and Moving Forward

Clinicians and other practitioners who pursue this brainstorming exercise will identify more ideas for positive change than can be implemented with available time and resources. An important next step is to choose the 10 best improvement ideas from the current list and then to narrow this list again to the top five most powerful (and plausible) ideas.

This narrowing of the list can be accomplished through a process of "multivoting" (as discussed in such resources as *The Team Handbook,* by Scholtes, Joiner, and Streibel[8]). If, for example, five team members are working on the current project, and 60 initial improvement ideas have been generated, then each participant receives 15 votes (that is, one-fourth of 60) during a first round of selection. Individuals choose from the initial list of 15 improvement ideas on the basis of criteria such as (a) largest potential impact, (b) easiest to accomplish—least costly in terms of time and special resource(s), and (c) easiest to test quickly. The ideas with most votes are retained for a second round of selection, following group discussion based on the aforementioned criteria. A third and fourth round follow as needed. During each cycle, each

participant receives the number of votes approximately equal to one-fourth of the remaining ideas. This process of sequential voting and discussing can quickly generate consensus on five most promising improvement ideas for actual testing.

By confronting initial challenges to change and by exploring local sources of information already available to most clinical practices (including staff and patient expertise, internal and external collections of data, and reflective assessment of process dynamics), a large list of specific improvement ideas can been generated, and from this list a smaller set of the most achievable ideas can been defined. With this list in mind, we are ready to develop specific improvement strategies that will improve clinical value through attention to identified targets. In the next chapter, to support development of these strategies, we introduce the Clinical Improvement Worksheet, a powerful tool that facilitates translation of improvement ideas into specific action plans.

Use this workbook area to summarize and to reflect on your efforts in this chapter.

Our summary list of improvement ideas includes:

1. _____
2. _____
3. _____
4. _____
5. _____
6. _____
7. _____
8. _____
9. _____
10. _____

Our five most powerful improvement ideas are:

1. _____
2. _____
3. _____
4. _____
5. _____

References

1. Ruskin J.: *The Complete Works of John Ruskin.* New York City: Kelmscott Society, 1900, as found in http://www.quotationspage.com/quote/5219.html.
2. Roberts H. V., Sergesketter B. F.: *Quality Is Personal: A Foundation for Total Quality Management.* New York City: Free Press, 1993.
3. Institute for Clinical Systems Improvement: *Guidelines & More.* http://www.icsi.org/guidelines_and_more/ (accessed May 23, 2007).
4. Nelson E.C., et al.: Publicly reporting comprehensive quality and cost data: A health care system's transparency initiative. *Jt Comm J Qual Patient Saf* 31:573–584, Oct. 2005.
5. Dartmouth Medical School, Center for the Evaluative Clinical Sciences: *The Dartmouth Atlas of Health Care.* http://www.dartmouthatlas.org/index.shtm (accessed May 23, 2007).
6. De Bono E.: *Serious Creativity: Using the Power of Lateral Thinking to Create New Ideas.* New York City: HarperBusiness, 1992.
7. Langley G.J., Nolan K.M., Nolan T.W.: The foundation of improvement. *Quality Progress* 27:81–86, Jun. 1994.
8. Scholtes P.R., Joiner B.L., Streibel B.J.: *The Team Handbook: How to Use Teams to Improve Quality,* 3rd ed. Madison, WI: Oriel Incorporated, 2003.

Improving Clinical Care: A Clinical Improvement Worksheet

Eugene C. Nelson, Paul B. Batalden, Stephen K. Plume, Julie K. Johnson, Joel S. Lazar

Every system is perfectly designed to get the results it gets. —Paul B. Batalden[1]

Improvement in clinical microsystems proceeds in a manner analogous to patient care itself; both endeavors build on cycles of goal clarification, assessment, intervention, and reassessment. Reflective practitioners of clinical improvement set their aim on specific targets in the caregiving process, clarify these processes through careful analysis, and implement measurable tests of change. Monitoring the outcomes of these interventions permits further refinement of initial goals and of the interventions themselves. Small tests of change can be conducted in everyday clinical practice, enabling individual providers and entire health care teams to learn from and to improve on their work.

In this chapter we introduce the Clinical Improvement Worksheet, a practical and flexible tool that supports the improvement of patient care in real-world settings. After defining and analyzing a core clinical process in some detail, we review specific steps in the redesign of this process and discuss strategies for testing the impact of redesign on both quality and costs. We explore the improvement worksheet's facilitation of practice-based learning and improvement in a detailed case study, and conclude with some general observations on the process of change itself.

As emphasized in Chapter 1, improvement work is the responsibility of all health professionals. This does not imply, however, that all improvement efforts must be implemented in a similar manner. Indeed, some initiatives are best pursued by a single practitioner, whereas others benefit from the active engagement of multiple clinical and nonclinical staff. (*See* Sidebar 3-1, page 26, for further discussion of this topic.) In this chapter, we use the Clinical Improvement Worksheet to focus

specifically on team-based initiatives. In Appendix A (pages 135–155), readers can find a modified improvement worksheet that has been adapted for use by individual practitioners.

In addition, although we emphasize (in this and other chapters) the development of quality initiatives to improve specific clinical outcomes, we also recognize the value of interventions whose impact on patient care is less direct. Nonclinical processes are important targets for quality innovation, and in Sidebar 3-2 (page 27) we consider appropriate strategies for improvement work in this domain.

The Core Clinical Process

Every episode of care begins with identification of a patient need, continues for short or long durations of time, and might involve multiple patient-clinician encounters in either ambulatory or inpatient settings (or both). Close attention to the structure of these clinical encounters enables us to target specific processes for practice-based improvement.

Each care-seeking episode has three phases: before, during, and after. In most cases, the process begins when a community-dwelling person experiences a new need for health care services such as diagnosis, prevention, treatment, or rehabilitation. Before initiation of the care-seeking episode itself, this individual already has a clinical (or biological) and a functional status, both of which can be assessed and monitored over time. The care seeker also has expectations to be satisfied and a history of costs associated with this particular clinical need. For example, most people have expectations about the way care should be delivered and a set of desired or "hoped for" health outcomes on the basis

SIDEBAR 3-1. Individual and Team Improvement

Although improvement work is the responsibility of all health care professionals, some well-intentioned clinicians are deterred by the common emphasis on team-based models to support this work. Many ideas are generated through the multidisciplinary perspectives of an improvement team and are supported and sustained by the interactions, skills, and buy-in of diverse members. However, not all decisions and actions are best made by committee, and the dynamics of group process can be time-consuming and sometimes counterproductive.

In fact, both individual and group models of clinical improvement are appropriate (and necessary!) to optimize quality and value in the varied contexts of real-world clinical care. The best size for an improvement team will depend on local resources (human and material) and on the task itself. Both solo and group improvement activities can be further subdivided as follows:

True solo improvement work can be performed by anyone at any time, but individuals can also participate in action-learning groups convened by a local leader. In a setting analogous to the "quality circle" used by Toyota and other high-

performing manufacturing companies, individuals proceed with their own projects at their own pace but receive regular feedback and support from colleagues who are also testing improvements in their everyday jobs.

At the more formal group level, improvements can be tested by small numbers of people from one's own work group, often with input from participants who serve in complementary, interdisciplinary roles. Alternatively, small teams can be drawn together from different work groups (or clinical units) that are based in different parts of the organization, or that support different steps in the care continuum. This latter model is employed quite commonly by health care organizations to implement targeted improvement projects.

Improvement work need not be restricted to special quality improvement teams that meet at special times. Instead, a more inclusive understanding of improvement opportunities permits nuanced integration of such work into everyone's daily routines, and it also supports synchronization and development of new resources that are beyond the reach of individuals.

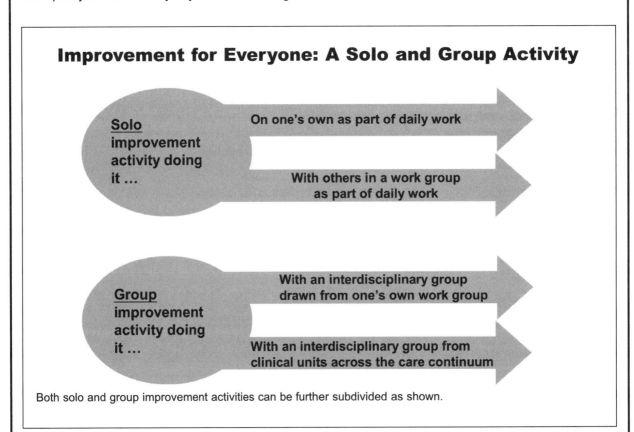

Improvement for Everyone: A Solo and Group Activity

Solo improvement activity doing it ...
- On one's own as part of daily work
- With others in a work group as part of daily work

Group improvement activity doing it ...
- With an interdisciplinary group drawn from one's own work group
- With an interdisciplinary group from clinical units across the care continuum

Both solo and group improvement activities can be further subdivided as shown.

SIDEBAR 3-2. **Clinical and Nonclinical Process Improvements**

There are countless quality, safety, and cost improvements to be made in every health care delivery system. As we emphasize in the present chapter, and in this book overall, many such improvements are targeted specifically to patient care outcomes—clinical, functional, satisfaction, costs—in a direct and substantial way. The Clinical Improvement Worksheet supports improvement work in precisely these domains.

However, nonclinical processes are also important targets for quality innovation. Improvements of this sort might have direct impact on patient outcomes, although they might enhance patient experience or clinical service indirectly. So, for example, improvements in the accuracy and timeliness of medical record transcription, or in the quality of food for hospitalized patients, or in the reporting time for diagnostic laboratory results, can be key targets for process improvement in health care settings. Other interventions (such as improved equity and access, or streamlining of administrative processes) might indeed impact patient outcomes downstream, although in a manner that is not easily measurable in the short term.

Many modern improvement methods are easily adapted for use in these situations. Two of the best known general process improvement models are the Define, Measure, Analyze, Improve, and Control (DMAIC) system used in Six Sigma programs[1] and the plan-do-study-act (PDSA) approach.[2,3] These valuable, general models can be used for practice-based learning and clinical improvement. Although these general models are less specific to clinical care and to patient-oriented outcomes, they have the advantage of adaptability to any improvement context that might support health care service delivery (such as medical records, pharmacy, or human resources). See Appendix A for the generic PDSA-SDSA (standardize-do-study-act) Worksheet, which supports improvement work of any type.

References

1. George M., et al.: *The Lean Six Sigma Pocket Toolbook*. New York City: McGraw Hill, 2005.
2. Deming W.E.: *Out of the Crisis*. Cambridge, MA: Massachusetts Institute of Technology Center for Advanced Engineering Study, 1986.
3. Langley G.J., et al.: *The Improvement Guide: A Practical Approach to Enhancing Organizational Performance*. San Francisco: Jossey-Bass Publishers, 1996.

---

of their symptoms and own prior experience or the experience of others. In addition, people incur both direct and indirect costs that are related to the needs that bring them in for care. Over a lifetime, these costs accumulate and create a longitudinal cost profile that derives from accumulated experiences and utilization of health care resources. (*See* our discussion of the Clinical Value Compass, initiated in Chapter 1 and elaborated in Chapter 4.)

When the health need is sufficiently compelling, it commonly prompts an individual to access the health care delivery system. On entry into this system, the individual is labeled traditionally as a *patient,* though other terms such as *customer* or *care seeker* have also been applied. Regardless of the chosen language, this person now becomes a participant in the core clinical process, and (importantly) becomes a beneficiary of services that clinicians and clinical team members provide. These services are in fact the sequence of actions that constitute the

core clinical process. They are depicted in Figure 3-1 (page 28) and can be characterized by the following specific activities:

- **Patient assessment**, on the basis of data collection from history taking, physical examination, and diagnostic tests
- **Diagnosis and classification** of the patient's need, on the basis of integration of pertinent information from the aforementioned assessment
- **Treatment regimen**, on the basis of clinical diagnosis, and individualized to specific preferences and priorities of this patient
- **Follow-up monitoring** of the patient and patient's needs over time

The quality and costs of care can be analyzed in terms of the impact of that care on clinical status, functional status and well-being, satisfaction, and costs. Again, the

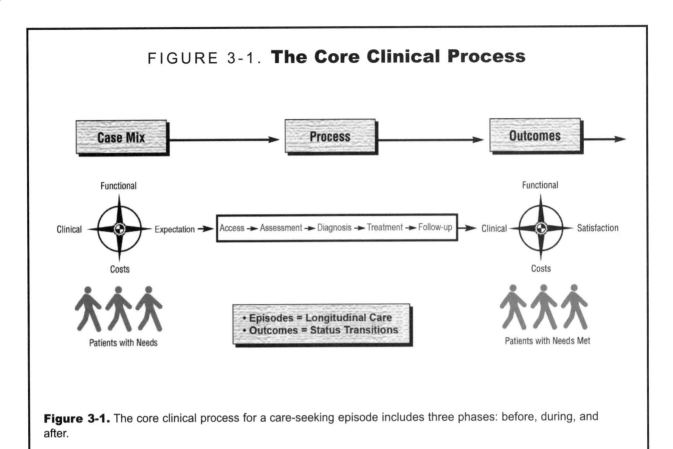

FIGURE 3-1. **The Core Clinical Process**

Figure 3-1. The core clinical process for a care-seeking episode includes three phases: before, during, and after.

Clinical Value Compass provides a framework for monitoring changes in these outcomes over time, and in Chapter 4 we explore this value compass–based monitoring process in greater detail. As noted in Figure 3-1 (above), these health outcomes are really health transitions. Living systems (including individual patients in their biological, social, and economic contexts) are dynamic rather than static entities, and are best characterized in terms of ongoing change. The practitioner's challenge is to take action so that each patient experiences the most favorable health transitions in the most satisfying and least costly manner. The case example in Sidebar 3-3 (page 29) illustrates the core clinical process involved in surgical correction of carpal tunnel syndrome (CTS).

The Clinical Improvement Worksheet

How can the improvement of clinical work be incorporated into busy doctors' offices and hospital routines without disrupting the smooth delivery of care? And how can this improvement be promoted in a manner that builds on clinicians' professional values of science and healing, their intrinsic curiosity about cause and effect, and their personal desire to find the best way to care for their patients?

The Clinical Improvement Worksheet, shown in Figure 3-2 (page 30) and Figure 3-3 (page 34), is a simple tool designed to facilitate frontline practitioners' blending of clinical improvement work with core processes of actual patient care. Based on a sequential model of quality innovation,[2] the improvement worksheet guides providers through self-assessment of caregiving processes, facilitates application of local knowledge in the development of small pilot tests of change, and directs attention to measures of both health outcomes and cost reduction.

Side A (Figure 3-2) of the improvement worksheet blends improvement thinking with the core clinical process in a manner that practitioners can easily tailor to their own patient care routines. Side B (Figure 3-3) invites more focused attention to the development and implementation of specific tests of change in clinical settings. The methods condensed in this improvement worksheet derive from extensive clinical experiences in myriad improvement and innovation contexts. Our own experience confirms that this graphic and flexible tool offers practitioners a simple format to visualize clinical and improvement processes, to record progress, and to share work in a standardized manner.

In the section that follows, we walk through the Clinical Improvement Worksheet and thus through the

---

SIDEBAR 3-3. **Case Example: The Core Clinical Process**

Tim, a 43-year-old computer systems analyst and avid tennis player, calls his primary care physician, Dr. Clark, on a Sunday night, complaining of severe hand and wrist pain. He tells Dr. Clark that this pain has progressed during the preceding six months, and is now quite severe. Tim thinks that more aggressive intervention might be required than the medication, splints, and physical therapy that have already been administered. The next morning during Tim's office visit, Dr. Clark takes a brief history, performs a directed physical examination, and concludes that the exacerbation represents further progression of carpal tunnel syndrome. He refers Tim to his colleague, Dr. Valiant, for consultation regarding surgery, because prior conservative treatment has failed. Dr. Valiant sees Tim a few days later, confirms the diagnosis, recommends surgery, and schedules the surgical procedure for two weeks later in the first available slot.

On the appointed day, Tim and his wife go to the hospital at 7:00 A.M. to prepare for surgery that had been scheduled for 9:00 A.M., but which is now pushed back to 11:00 A.M. because of higher-priority emergency cases. At 11:30 A.M., Tim undergoes a carpal tunnel release procedure under general anesthesia. He is discharged at 3:30 P.M. with instructions to visit Dr. Valiant's office in a few days for a brief wound-healing check with the clinical assistant, to schedule a follow-up appointment in four weeks, and to call if he experiences trouble during the next week.

Tim's wife drives him home (she has taken the day off from teaching to be with her husband). Tim feels a little weak from the anesthesia effects and stays home from work for the next two days. He returns to work the next Monday but experiences limitations on the job: He can't comfortably use his computer keyboard for extended periods of time.

At the four-week follow-up visit, Dr. Valiant

asks Tim how he is doing. He learns that Tim still suffers some hand symptoms (pain and tingling with no numbness) but has begun using his computer again. When Tim asks when he can resume playing tennis, the doctor informs him that, with some physical therapy and time, he will most likely be able to return to his game in several months. On his way out, Tim states that he is fairly happy with the surgery results and that he really appreciates Dr. Valiant's care but that he wishes that his recovery would proceed more quickly. Taking time off from work and then experiencing limitations upon returning to work have put him way behind on a big project. He tells Dr. Valiant that he appreciates his friendly, down-to-earth manner and his genuine concern, and he believes that, from a technical point of view, the surgeon and staff did a great job. Tim is glad, however, that he doesn't have to foot the bill, because the whole procedure was much more costly than he had expected.

Tim roughly estimates the total cost of his care to be almost $4,000. Dr. Valiant is surprised at this high figure, and asks Tim to break the costs down. Tim's estimates included the following:
- Physician office visits: $150
- Surgical fees: $1,140
- Hospital facility charge: $800
- Anesthesia: $320
- Laboratory test charges: $250
  — Total medical care charges: $2,660
- Tim's three days out of work: $900
- Tim's wife's one day lost from work: $200 (to be with Tim during surgery)
- Substitute teacher cost: $150
  — Total time lost from work: $1,250
  — Total Cost: $3,910

Following this encounter, Dr. Valiant begins to consider new approaches to carpal tunnel release that might be faster, better, and cheaper.

---

generic steps of practice-based improvement work itself. We then demonstrate the improvement worksheet's utility in one real-world application, and we invite readers to envision and to experiment with their own local applications. A recent modification of the improvement worksheet and the complete Clinical Improvement Worksheet user's manual are included in Appendix A.

Team Up

As described above, and elaborated in Sidebar 3.1, some improvement efforts are best pursued by a single practitioner, whereas other improvement efforts benefit from the active engagement of multiple clinical and nonclinical staff. When a collective approach is felt to be most appropriate, core participants must consider, early in the endeavor, who has greatest knowledge of the clinical process and who should be invited to join the improvement team. This team might be a natural work group of people who practice together on a daily basis, such as a primary care or obstetrical team, or it might be an ad hoc group brought together to improve management of a specific clinical concern, such as urinary tract infection or total joint replacement. Realistically, not all team members can be selected until specific target populations are identified and until the broad aim of an improvement project is clarified. As the improvement team is developed, the following guidelines should be considered:

- Select individuals who are familiar with different elements of the core process.
- Select individuals from different disciplines to reflect diverse areas of expertise and knowledge.
- Designate a leader who is credible and responsible for the technical process that needs improvement.
- Limit the number of members to eight or fewer.

- Choose an experienced team facilitator if participants are new to the improvement process.

Ready...Aim...

Side A of the Clinical Improvement Worksheet (Figure 3-2, below) poses four questions pertinent to the core clinical process and to its ongoing improvement:

1. Outcomes: What is the general aim of this work, and who are we trying to help?
2. Process: What is the process for giving care to this type of patient?
3. Changes: What ideas do we have for changing what is done (the process) to get better results?
4. Pilot: How can we pilot test an improvement idea?

Working through Side A provides a high-level view of the core clinical process, directing participants to get ready for change in general and empowering them to take aim at specific targets in the caregiving process. Attention will

---

FIGURE 3-2. **Clinical Improvement Worksheet, Side A**

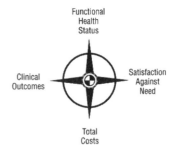

Clinical Improvement Worksheet
Aim: Accelerate clinical improvement by linking outcomes measurements and process knowledge with the design and conduct of pilot tests of change.

MEASUREMENT
Outcome   Outcome
Process   PDSA
PROCESS

② PROCESS ➡ **Analyze the process**
What's the process for giving care to this type of patient?

Patient with need for "x" → Access System → Assessment → Diagnosis → Treatment → Follow-Up →

① OUTCOMES ➡ **Select a population**
What's the general aim? Given our wish to limit/reduce the illness burden for "this type" of patient, what are the desired results?

Functional Health Status
Clinical Outcomes
Satisfaction Against Need
Total Costs

③ CHANGES ➡ **Generate change ideas**
What ideas do we have for changing what's done (process) to get better results?
• • •

④ PILOT ➡ **Select first/next change for pilot testing**
How can we pilot test an improvement idea using the PDSA (plan-do-study-act) method?

Figure 3-2. Side A of the Clinical Improvement Worksheet blends improvement thinking with the core clinical process. Copyright 1995, Trustees of Dartmouth College, Nelson, Batalden.

Using one clinical improvement idea from Chapter 2, develop an aim statement.

Clinical Improvement Worksheet

Aim: _____

_____

---

be focused on high-leverage areas for tests of change and will occur in a context that supports discussion of care processes and desired outcomes. On the basis of brainstorming work performed in Chapter 2, clinicians might already have a good idea of where improvement efforts should be focused.

1. Outcomes → Select a Population

What's the general aim? Identify a patient population in which there is both strong clinician interest and compelling organization need. Potential criteria include procedures or diagnoses with high volume, high cost (including long lengths of stay), high per-case improvement potential, tough market competition, and high probability of achieving change. Another important consideration is the perceived relevance of this improvement to patients, clinicians, and other stakeholders.

What are the desired results? State the aim in terms of the specific population selected. What results does the team hope to achieve, and how will it reduce the burden of illness for the target population? Start with a broad statement of the aim, and then focus it on the selected patient population.

Define the Population

On the basis of the general aim statement, brainstorm to identify potentially important clinical, functional, satisfaction, and cost outcomes for the selected patient population. Start with clinical outcomes ("west" on the Clinical Value Compass), proceed to functional ("north") and satisfaction ("east"), and finish with costs ("south").

2. Process → Analyze the Process

What's the process for giving care to this type of patient? Construct a flowchart of the care-delivery process. Begin by specifying the process boundaries, that is, the steps where this core clinical process starts and fin-

ishes for the selected patient population. Specifically define the following:

1. The process starts when patients _____. (fill in the blank).
2. The process ends when patients _____. (fill in the blank).

Draft a flowchart of the delivery process by talking through the specific points of action, decision, and transition that characterize a typical patient encounter. Confirm and modify impressions by physically walking through actual steps, as these might be experienced by the patient. Begin with a simple high-level flowchart (5 to 20 steps), and refine it over time.

Specify the patient characteristics that are likely to affect processes of care delivery or that alter the probability of specific patient outcomes. Descriptors that tend to influence processes or outcomes include patient demographics (age, gender, education), health parameters (diagnosis, severity of primary diagnosis, comorbidity), and patient preferences (treatment expectations, lifestyle choices, and valuation of specific results).

3. Changes → Generate Change Ideas

What ideas do we have for changing what's done (the process) to get better results? Think about the aim, the desired results (clinical, functional, satisfaction, costs), and the delivery process (as represented in a flowchart). Brainstorm as many changes as possible that could improve care or lower costs. Clarify the concepts and combine those that are redundant. Determine the most promising change idea for pilot testing.

4. Pilot → Select Change for Pilot Testing

How can we pilot test an improvement idea? Because not all changes lead to improvement, innovations must be tested to assure that they add value to the core clinical

Define your population.

OUTCOMES ➡ Select a population
What's the general aim? Given our wish to limit/reduce the illness burden for "this type" of patient, what are the desired results?

_____

_____

_____

Identify important outcomes for that population.

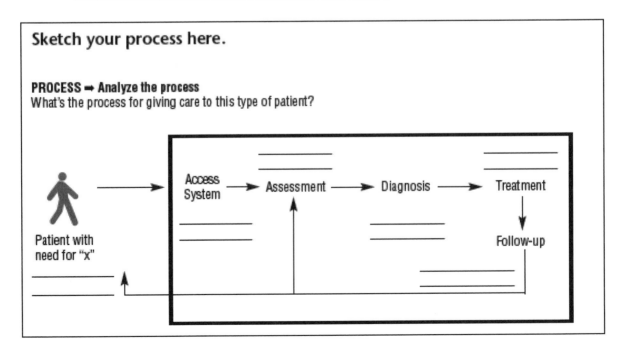

Sketch your process here.

PROCESS ➡ Analyze the process
What's the process for giving care to this type of patient?

What are the most promising changes?

CHANGES → **Generate change ideas**

What ideas do we have for changing what's done (process) to get better results?

_____

_____

_____

---

process. A simple before-and-after study design can support the assessment of specific change ideas. Ask whether, and how, participants can pilot test one idea using the PDSA (Plan-Do-Study-Act) method. If possible, the best tests of change are performed quickly and on a small scale. Now is the time to identify logistical, political, or timing issues that might support or hinder the pilot test's implementation.

Aim...Fire...Hit (or Miss)

Side B of the Clinical Improvement Worksheet (Figure 3-3, page 34) focuses further attention on a specific test of change. It facilitates clarification of an improvement objective and then guides the team through specific action steps in the PDSA cycle.

The left-hand side of this improvement worksheet invites participants to reflect on the composition of their team and on specific aims, measures, and characteristics of the selected change. Individually, and in conference with team members, consider the following questions:

1. Who should work on this improvement?
2. What are we trying to accomplish?
3. How will we know whether a change is an improvement?

4. How would you describe the change that you have selected for testing?
5. How shall we *plan* the pilot?
6. What are we learning as we *do* the pilot?
7. As we *study* what happened, what have we learned?
8. As we *act* to hold the gains or abandon our pilot efforts, what needs to be done?

Team Members → Who Should Work on This Improvement?

From the original group identified, or among other individuals not previously considered, who needs to be directly involved in this work, and who does not? Use the improvement worksheet to refine thinking about who is needed on the team. Identify team members, and choose an appropriate leader. Participants might also wish to name a facilitator, record keeper, and timekeeper, whose roles can rotate from meeting to meeting. Ancillary team resources should be identified as well, including administrators and coaches, who coordinate or serve as improvement resources across several teams and improvement efforts. See Sidebar 3-4 (page 35) for further discussion of team formation and effective team meetings.

What will your pilot test be?

PILOT → **Select first/next change for pilot testing**

How can we pilot test an improvement idea using the PDSA (Plan-Do-Study-Act) method?

_____

_____

_____

FIGURE 3-3. **Clinical Improvement Worksheet, Side B**

Making Improvements: Clinical Improvement Worksheet

TEAM MEMBERS →Who should work on this improvement?

1. _Leader_   5. _____
2. _Facilitator_ 6. _____
3. _____   7. _____
4. _____   8. _____

Coach _____

Administrative
Support _____

(A) **SPECIFIC AIM →What are we trying to accomplish?**
(more specific _aim_)

(B) **MEASURES →How will we know whether a change is an improvement?**

(C) **SELECTED CHANGE →How would you describe the change that you have selected for testing?**

(D) **PLAN →How shall we _plan_ the pilot?**
• Who? Does what? When? With what tools and training?

• Baseline data to be collected?

(E) **DO →What are we learning as we _do_ the pilot?**

(F) **STUDY →As we _study_ what happened, what have we learned?**
• Did original outcomes improve?

(G) **ACT →As we _act_ to hold the gains or abandon our pilot efforts, what needs to be done?**

Figure 3-3. Side B of the Clinical Improvement Worksheet invites more focused attention to the development and implementation of specific tests of change in clinical settings. Copyright 1995, Trustees of Dartmouth College, Nelson, Batalden.

Fill in the team leader, facilitator (if there is one), and team members. Also keep track of any ancillary members who might support the work of the team.

TEAM MEMBERS → Who should work on this improvement?

1. Leader _____   5. _____

2. Facilitator _____   6. _____

3. _____   7. _____

4. _____   8. _____

Coach _____   Administrative Support _____

Ⓐ A Specific Aim → What Are We Trying to Accomplish?

What specifically is the team trying to accomplish with this test of change? Make a more definite and structured aim statement that clarifies intentions, expectations, and priorities. This aim will guide subsequent planning and self-assessment of the proposed pilot study.

To help sharpen the aim statement, complete the following sentences:

1. The aim is to improve the quality and value of _____ (fill in name of clinical care process).
2. This clinical care process starts with _____ (fill in starting point of the process) and the process ends when _____ (fill in end point of the process).
3. By working on this process, we expect that _____ (fill in the anticipated better outcomes).
4. It is important to work on this process now because _____ (insert reasons that make this important from the perspective of the patient, clinician, or purchaser of care).

Now define the specific aim.

SPECIFIC AIM → What are we trying to accomplish?
(More specific aim)

_____
_____
_____
_____

SIDEBAR 3-4. Improvement Team Meeting Process and Holding Effective Meetings

Because time is a precious resource for practitioners of clinical improvement, efficient and effective team meetings will optimize the active and intelligent participation of all team members. Leaders of such groups might wish to educate themselves in the principles and methods of team formation, team function, and productive and enjoyable team meetings. Much has been written on this topic. We recommend *The Team Handbook*, by Scholtes, Joiner, and Streibel,[1] as an excellent resource. Further information on effective meetings and team meeting roles can be found at http://www.clinicalmicrosystem.org.

Reference
1. Scholtes P.R., Joiner B.L., Streibel B.J.: *The Team Handbook: How to Use Teams to Improve Quality*, 3rd ed. Madison, WI: Oriel Incorporated, 2003.

Ⓑ Measures → How Will We Know Whether a Change Is an Improvement?

A few balanced measures can be used to evaluate the success (outcomes and costs) of the pilot. Measures should flow from the specific aim statement cited in Step A (directly left) and from the more general, higher-level list of outcomes generated in Step 1 on Worksheet Side A.

What specifically will we measure and how?

MEASURES → How will we know whether a change is an improvement?

_____

_____

_____

_____

Ⓒ Selected Change → How Would We Describe the Change Selected for Testing?

Describe the change that has been selected for testing, and (important!) use this spot on the improvement worksheet to keep track of other potential changes the team might wish to try in the future. The essence of continual improvement is to run repeated, rapid, and increasingly effective tests of change.

Describe the change selected.

SELECTED CHANGE → How would we describe the change selected for testing?

_____

_____

_____

_____

PDSA Cycle

The basic steps of a PDSA improvement cycle are elaborated in the right-hand column of the improvement worksheet's Side B. Having taken aim at a specific improvement target, team members are empowered in the PDSA cycle to fire more accurately and to determine whether their shot was a hit or a miss. The cycle challenges participants to address (through action) the following essential questions:

1. How shall we _plan_ the pilot?
2. What are we learning as we _do_ the pilot?
3. As we _study_ what happened, what have we learned?
4. As we _act_ to hold the gains or abandon our pilot efforts, what needs to be done?

Ⓓ Plan → How Shall We _Plan_ the Pilot?

Who? Does what? When? With what tools and training? Write a brief change protocol that answers these questions and then illustrate the protocol with a simple flowchart. A good plan must be executed well to succeed; participants involved should know what they are doing and why they are doing it. Flowchart illustrations can be beneficial here.

Baseline data to be collected: Write a brief data collection protocol indicating who will gather and analyze what data from what sources. Use precise operational definitions so that all participants speak the same language and enact the same protocol.

FIGURE 3-4. **Completed Clinical Improvement Worksheet: Carpal Tunnel Syndrome***

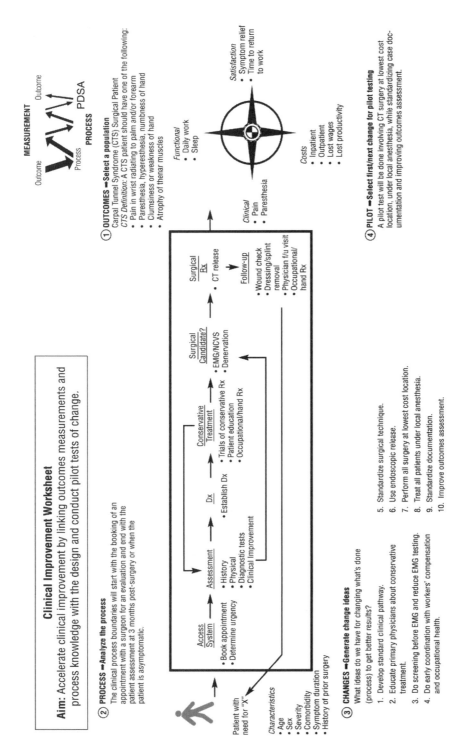

Figure 3-4. Side A of a completed Clinical Improvement Worksheet demonstrates progress made by the Carpal Tunnel Team.

* PDSA, Plan-Do-Study-Act; Dx, diagnosis; EMG, electromyography; f/u, follow-up; NCVS, nerve conduction velocity study; Rx, treatment.

What's the plan and how will it be implemented?

PLAN → How shall we *plan* the pilot?

• Who? Does what? When? With what tools and training?

_____

_____

_____

_____

• Baseline data to be collected:

_____

_____

_____

_____

Ⓔ Do → What Are We Learning as We *Do* the Pilot?

Keep a diary of the pilot project, open to reflections from all participants. Comment on whether discrete steps, and the intervention as a whole, are proceeding as planned. The results of this pilot will be no better than the care with which the planned change was executed. Observations about the process can help prepare the way for making more powerful changes in the future.

Keep track of how you're doing.

DO → What are we learning as we *do* the pilot?

_____

_____

_____

_____

Ⓕ Study → As We Study What Happened, What Have We Learned?

Did original outcomes improve? Analyze the pilot test results in a way that answers the main question: Did the change lead to the predicted improvement?

What results have we seen, and what do they mean?

STUDY → As we study what happened, what have we learned?

Did original outcomes improve?

_____

_____

_____

_____

Ⓖ Act → As We *Act* to Hold the Gains or Abandon Our Pilot Efforts, What Needs to Be Done?

If the pilot was successful, the next task is to incorporate this positive change into daily work routines, so that ongoing delivery of care proceeds efficiently and effectively. If the pilot was not successful, then analyze the source(s) of this failure, and welcome this new opportunity to learn. Failure is an invitation to generate new theories of cause and effect. Don't be discouraged. Many tests of change will fail to produce the desired positive result, but *all* such tests can stimulate insight that supports future, and perhaps more effective, clinical improvement.

> **Where do we take this from here?**
>
> **ACT →** As we *act* to hold the gains or abandon our pilot efforts, what needs to be done?
>
> _____
> _____
> _____
> _____

Using the Clinical Improvement Worksheet: Case Study on Improving Carpal Tunnel Surgery

The orthopedic surgical section chief in Dartmouth-Hitchcock Clinic's southern region had a strong interest in clinical improvement and outcomes measurement, and he wished to acquire hands-on experience. He thus developed the Carpal Tunnel Team, whose work is documented in the following discussion. Figure 3-4 (page 37) shows a completed Side A of the Carpal Tunnel Team's Clinical Improvement Worksheet, highlighting the team's efforts. Our account of this case follows the structure of the improvement worksheet itself.

Team Members → Who should work on this improvement?

The Carpal Tunnel Team consisted of five surgeons, one hand therapist (added later), one nurse, two managers, one statistician, one coach, and one team facilitator. To begin, participants agreed to schedule two-hour meetings every other week, to follow structured meeting agendas, and to designate specific roles of leader, timekeeper, recorder, and facilitator.

① Outcomes → Select a Population (Meeting 1)

After considering several surgical conditions where care might be locally improved, team participants selected carpal tunnel syndrome (CTS) as the target for focused attention. CTS is a high-volume problem that significantly affects both patients and employers. Indeed, it was (and remains) one of the three most common surgical procedures performed by this surgical group. Current care is expensive, although failure to treat also has occupational and economic consequences. Many aspects of the process and its outcomes are easily measured, and the optimal management strategy is not controversial among participating surgeons. Thus, the clinical team identified a high-volume patient population with a well-defined need, for whom intervention was likely to yield worthwhile improvement.

What's the general aim? The team was formed to improve outcomes and to reduce costs for CTS patients and simultaneously to increase "improvement capacity" itself through practice with formal improvement methodologies.

Given our wish to limit or to reduce the illness burden for this type of patient, what are the desired results? The team brainstormed desirable outcomes for each of the four Clinical Value Compass points and then reduced the list (by sequential multivoting) to identify the two most important measures for each value compass point. The final results included the following:

- Clinical outcomes: pain, paresthesia
- Functional health status: daily work ability, sleep

- Satisfaction: perceived symptom relief, satisfaction with time to return to work
- Costs: inpatient charges and outpatient charges, lost wages, and lost productivity

A CTS Clinical Value Compass annotated with selected measures was created on a flip chart. The CTS Clinical Value Compass flip chart page was displayed at each subsequent meeting to help maintain focus (Figure 3-5, below).

② Process → Analyze the Process (Meeting 2)

What's the process for giving care to this type of patient? The team represented the CTS care delivery process on a flowchart. This was done by establishing an arbitrary start and end point and by asking each team member to write on adhesive notes simple phrases that described his or her work for each point in the core delivery process. All notes were displayed on a visible flip chart; the team organized these notes into a logical progression and then analyzed the resultant flowchart. Refinements were made through addition of missed steps and elimination of redundancies.

The team then broke into two groups: one to define patient characteristics that affected processes and outcomes (such as age, sex, severity, comorbidity, symptom duration, history of surgery), and the other to construct an agreed-on operational definition for the CTS patient who consulted a participating surgeon (this definition is shown on the team's improvement worksheet in Figure 3-4, page 37, under "Outcomes").

③ Changes → Generate Change Ideas (Meeting 3)

What ideas do we have for changing what's done (process) to get better results? The team reviewed the general aim, the CTS Clinical Value Compass measures, the operational definitions, and the current clinical processes. Next, team members took five minutes to think on their own (in silent idea generation) about changes that could be made—either small adjustments or large innovations—to produce better results. These ideas for change were shared, the list was clarified, and the team multi-voted to select a change for pilot testing. (The original list is shown in Figure 3-4, page 37.)

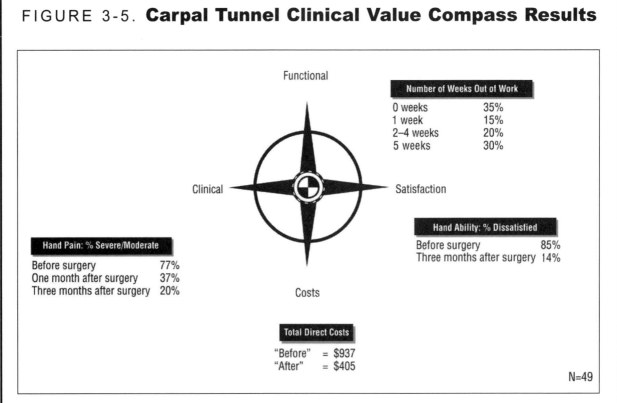

FIGURE 3-5. **Carpal Tunnel Clinical Value Compass Results**

Number of Weeks Out of Work	
0 weeks	35%
1 week	15%
2–4 weeks	20%
5 weeks	30%

Hand Ability: % Dissatisfied	
Before surgery	85%
Three months after surgery	14%

Hand Pain: % Severe/Moderate	
Before surgery	77%
One month after surgery	37%
Three months after surgery	20%

Total Direct Costs		
"Before"	=	$937
"After"	=	$405

N=49

Figure 3-5. Selected results are shown on the Clinical Value Compass for the improvements implemented by the Carpal Tunnel Team.

④ Pilot → Select a Change for Pilot Testing (Meeting 4)

How can we pilot test an improvement idea using the PDSA method? The team selected two main ideas to combine in a single pilot test:

1. Perform the carpal tunnel release (CTR) surgical procedure under local anesthesia.
2. Perform the CTR procedure at the lowest-cost location.

The team recognized that while this change was being tested, adoption of two further change ideas would be essential:

3. Standardize documentation.
4. Improve assessment of patient outcomes.

Team members agreed that a test of change was practicable in all three locations, and by all participating surgeons. The group hypothesized that this change would result in greater patient satisfaction and lower costs (direct and indirect) to patients, employers, and the delivery system.

Ⓐ Aim → What Are We Trying to Accomplish? (Meeting 4)

The team sharpened its aim statement to the following:

> Our aim is to improve our care of patients with CTS and to improve our ability to study clinical processes. This clinical process begins with the presentation of the patient to the surgical specialist and ends 12 weeks after the procedure or when a patient is asymptomatic, whichever is later. Our plan is to see if surgical patients treated with local anesthesia in a low-cost location for their carpal tunnel release have superior satisfaction with care, comparable clinical and functional outcomes, and lower medical (and social) costs.

Ⓑ Measures → How Will We Know That a Change Is an Improvement? (Meeting 4)

The team decided to develop operational definitions for selected measures related to clinical outcomes (such as pain, paresthesia), functioning (such as daily work, sleep), satisfaction (with such things as speed of recovery, convenience, or treatment timeliness), and costs (such as medical charges to patient, days lost from work).

Ⓒ Selected Change → How Would We Describe the Change That We Have Selected for Testing? (Meeting 4)

The team had generated a working list of possible changes (Side A, Step 3 of the improvement worksheet) in Meeting 3. Of the ideas listed in that section, the actual trial would include these changes:

*   Perform all surgery at the lowest-cost location.
*   Treat all patients under local anesthesia.
*   Standardize documentation of care.
*   Improve outcomes assessment.

To facilitate standardization and outcome assessment, new standardized assessments of patient case mix, treatment processes, and health outcomes were designed into the delivery process. Data were gathered from the patient and the surgeon (before surgery and 4 and 12 weeks after surgery) using self-coding data collection forms.

Ⓓ Plan → How Shall We *Plan* the Pilot? (Meetings 4–10)

Who? Does what? When? With what tools and training? The change was to be piloted in all three regional locations where CTR was performed. The team brainstormed a task list and then developed a critical pathway of steps to prepare for the pilot study. Some of these steps were as follows:

*   Set up and define measures.
*   Obtain cost estimates from potential outpatient surgical centers.

- Estimate cost for current system versus new system.
- Make detailed protocol using flowchart method.
- Determine budgetary implications of plan.
- Gain agreement from surgeons in all locations.
- Develop data-analysis plan and review relevant literature.
- Design self-coding data forms for use by patients and surgeons.
- Establish computer-based analysis system.
- Identify and purchase needed equipment.
- Determine plan for using surgical procedure room.
- Select and train staff to assist in new CTR method.
- Collect cost and utilization data on old method.
- Begin new method by conducting CTR in lowest-cost location, using local anesthesia and gathering standardized measures.

Baseline data to be collected: The team collected prospective data from both patients and surgeons. The patient data included measures of clinical status, functional status, satisfaction, and indirect costs associated with time lost from work. Data collected from surgeons included information on history, clinical status, the CTR procedure, surgical findings, and postoperative care. Information from patients was gathered from self-completed questionnaires at three points in time: before surgery, 4 weeks after surgery, and 12 weeks after surgery. Information from surgeons was obtained at these same time points, plus at the time of surgery. Great attention was given to construction of operational definitions for variables and to design of pre-coded questionnaires (for patients) and data collection forms (for surgeons), which could be used in real time with minimal interruption to care delivery. In the course of several drafts, these questionnaires and forms were color coded for ease of use. One person was identified to oversee the entire data collection process, from identification of patients who met CTR protocol criteria through collection of complete follow-up data.

Ⓔ Do → What Are We Learning as We *Do* the Pilot?

Early in the implementation of its actual pilot intervention, the Carpal Tunnel Team discovered that successful data collection at time of care delivery required modification of the initial protocol. The key to success was early review and detection of incomplete data collection forms, allowing the data coordinator to identify missing information. These forms could then be returned to clinicians and patients for timely completion, improving the quality of data collected. The team's experience with this "modification in progress" prompted scheduling of additional periodic reunions, the purpose of which was to monitor results of recently treated patients and to further adjust protocols as required.

Ⓕ Study → As We *Study* What Happened, What Have We Learned? Did Original Outcomes Improve?

To determine the impact of their first test of change (first PDSA cycle), the team analyzed results of its first 49 patients treated in the new protocol (that is, CTR performed at the lowest-cost location, under local anesthesia, and evaluated with standardized measurements over time). Data were collected on costs (old versus new method), and on patient-specific outcomes (clinical, functional, and satisfaction measurements before and after surgery). As illustrated on the Clinical Value Compass in Figure 3-5, page 40, and described below, specific outcomes improved, whereas costs decreased. Most notably, the following occurred:

- **Clinical.** The percentage of patients rating their hand pain as moderate or severe decreased from 77% before surgery to 37% at 4 weeks after surgery and to 20% at 12 weeks after surgery.
- **Functional.** Of the patients treated, 35% were able to return to work immediately, 15% returned in less than one week, 20% returned in two to four weeks, and 30% took five or more weeks.
- **Satisfaction.** Of the patients treated, 85% were dissatisfied with their ability to move their hand before surgery, and 14% were dissatisfied 12 weeks postoperatively. Patient satisfaction with local anesthesia was high (88%).
- **Costs.** Total direct costs for provision of care were reduced by more than 50%, from $937 to $405. These savings resulted from replacement of same-day inpatient surgery with ambulatory surgery under local anesthesia; elimina-

tion of preoperative appointment and ancillary tests; and elimination of handoffs from clinic to hospital for scheduling the procedure, transferring patient information, and transporting the patient. Because more than 70% of CTR procedures were prepaid, these reductions in costs were associated with better financial margins for this clinical activity.

These findings were gratifying but also suggested specific new targets for the second PDSA. In this next cycle, the team planned to address either upstream processes of presurgical screening (to simplify the identification of patients most likely to benefit from surgical treatment) or downstream disparities in functional outcome (to decrease time lost from work for the 30% of patients whose recovery was delayed).

Carpal Tunnel Team: Lessons Learned

The team learned several important lessons, the most important of which was that clinical improvement work is indeed fun and challenging. The team was energized by its initial work, and participants felt ready to move on to more challenging and costly areas of orthopedic work, such as total joint replacement.

The team also found that the pace of change is variable, even within a single project. The team moved rapidly through Side A of the improvement worksheet in only three weekly meetings, but slowed down considerably during the implementation phase, which required three months. Change can be fast, but not instantaneous; it is important not to be discouraged when slowdowns are encountered.

Although CTS was selected as a quick and noncontroversial opportunity for intervention, the team discovered that considerable effort was required to ensure clinician and staff support for the new method. As participants quickly appreciated, leaders of clinical change must facilitate and negotiate two forms of transition: process redesign (developing and testing a new way) and role redefinition (managing the human, political, and cultural dynamics that determine success or failure of the *new way* in the *old setting*).

The CTS team also learned to avoid potential extremes of data collection. Some earnest practitioners are at risk of jumping in to the intervention itself, without regard for quantitative assessment of that intervention's clinical or operational impact. Other individuals fall prey to the opposite problem and bog themselves down in excess measurement, to the potential detriment or disrup-

tion of patient care. Participants in more balanced interventions select a small number of carefully targeted measurements, with a preference for data that can be directly extracted from, or inserted into, the patient care process itself.

Overall, surgeons and staff learned that a relatively simple redesign of CTS care could yield higher clinical quality at significantly reduced cost. Indeed preliminary estimates suggest that charges to patients would be reduced substantially, by approximately $650 per case, and that patient time lost from work or normal routine would greatly decline. Use of surgeon time was expected to be more efficient as well, and operating margins for the delivery system were expected to shift from the prior *loss* of $90 per patient to a *profit* of more than $500 per patient. Although points on the Clinical Value Compass appear distinct during formal analysis and indeed seem to "pull" in opposite directions, our experience is that improvements in one domain almost always facilitate improvements in the others.

Carpal Tunnel Team: Limitations Observed

In every trial of clinical improvement, learning opportunities arise not only from successes but also from real or potential limitations. In the current case, for example, we can ask whether the Carpal Tunnel Team too quickly tested a change in clinical process—local anesthesia at lowest-cost location—without gathering baseline data on clinical, functional, and satisfaction outcomes. Certainly, a pre–post comparison in these domains would have been valuable, as it was in the assessment of cost. The real CTS team innovation, however, was the introduction of data monitoring itself: the care process was modified specifically to include real-time data collection on patient mix, treatment process, and outcomes, as reported by patients and clinicians themselves.

The team did seriously consider gathering baseline outcome data prior to initiating the clinical change. This option was eschewed, however, because of the following reasons:

- Baseline data collection would have delayed the test of change by several months.
- Anecdotal evidence from a local surgeon suggested that this practice change would be preferred by many patients (local anesthesia favored over general anesthesia).
- A reasonable alternate strategy was in place to initiate repeated tests of change (in an already changing

world), so that outcome data from change cycle 1 could serve as baseline data for change cycle 2.

Another potential criticism of the CTS process is the time spent in the project selection itself. Arguably, the changes selected for this initial improvement cycle were "no-brainers" that primarily targeted cost reductions. These changes might have been identified without the fuss and bother of team formation. A managed care plan, for example, could simply have mandated local anesthesia at the lowest-cost location, and this mandate might have reduced subsequent meeting and planning time.

This criticism has some at-face validity but neglects the important observation that successful change in clinical practice depends on genuine buy-in from physicians and staff. Improvement work is not a spectator sport. When clinicians feel ownership of change processes and innovations and particularly when they are the instigators and champions of such change, the initiatives are more likely to be accepted, and thus to promote more sustainable quality improvement.

Moving Forward

The Clinical Improvement Worksheet has been applied in ambulatory and inpatient settings to topics as diverse as primary prevention, acute surgical care, and posthospital rehabilitation. The instrument is useful whenever a specific clinical population can be identified that undergoes a more or less predictable clinical process. On the basis of experience with the improvement worksheet in these various contexts, we offer the following further recommendations for its effective use:

- **Think of ramping up improvements.** Improvement teams will benefit from conceptualizing their short-term work in longer-term contexts. Think about running repeated tests of change over time rather than finding the quick fix. Figure 3-6 (page 45) depicts a continual improvement ramp in which small (and rapid) tests of change support each other sequentially. A first test of change, for example, might be to standardize a single small step in a larger process that varies significantly. This might be followed by a second change in which the order of steps is modified so that delays are prevented downstream. A third change might be more substantial, such as the development of standing orders or care guidelines to clarify more generally the interventions that must occur during each stage of the process flow.

Each test is conducted to unsettle the existing sys-

tem and to provide useful information on the design of further change. With time, more and more trials are conducted, and the complexity of interventions might increase as experience with successful change accumulates. In this manner, a team might progress from simple, small improvements (with real but modest impact on quality and value) to total process redesign and radical reengineering (with a very large impact on quality and value). Participants often arrive at their first meeting with many ideas for improvement—these are usually the obvious changes. As the team ascends its ramp of sequential improvements, the breadth and depth of potential interventions expands in concert with increasing process knowledge itself.

- **Accelerate tests of change.** Although improvement work takes practice, the aim should be rapid redesign. With experience, both the number and the speed of change cycles can increase. Cutting cycle time (from conceptualization of the change concept to conclusion of a small-scale pilot test) should be a practice objective. Indeed, this cycle time can itself be the object of measurement, motivating teams to improve their very process of improvement. Setting an ambitious timetable early in the work can help to pick up the pace of change.

- **Think of multiple ways to make improvements.** The Clinical Improvement Worksheet is versatile. Question 3—"What ideas do we have for changing what's done to get better results?"—invites people to think broadly about change concepts that might produce better outcomes. As discussed more extensively in Chapter 6, a change concept is a general notion or approach to change that is useful in developing specific ideas for clinical improvement.[3] For example, if the change concept is "standardization," ideas for change might include development of clinical guidelines or design of a critical pathway.

Implementation in the Real World

Implementing changes in the real world can be challenging. Most of us suffer from "change-process illiteracy." We have only limited knowledge of how things really work in our own practices, and what we do know is not documented. This lack of knowledge of "what is" impedes our ability to design "what should be." To make matters worse, we often fail to understand and anticipate resistance to change among colleagues who must be involved (at the front line and in the front office) if clinical innovations are to be successful.

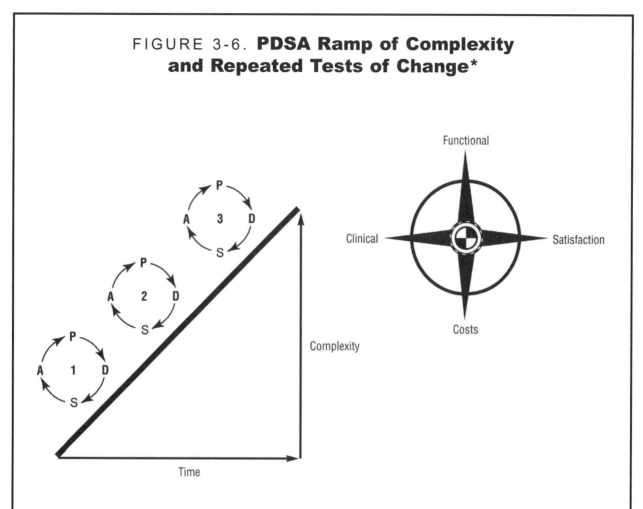

FIGURE 3-6. **PDSA Ramp of Complexity and Repeated Tests of Change***

Figure 3-6. A continual improvement ramp shows how implementing repeated tests of change allows an organization to improve quality and reduce costs over time, rather than attempting a quick fix.
* PDSA, Plan-Do-Study-Act.

Thus, to facilitate positive change in real-world clinical practice, improvement teams must maximize their understanding of current care processes, and leaders of improvement work must be especially skilled in managing the interpersonal dimensions of process change. We conclude the current chapter by addressing these two topics in turn.

Visualizing the Core Clinical Process

Improvement teams find great value in diagramming the core clinical process and then in addressing each component of this process in turn. As discussed previously, several generic activities proceed sequentially in all or most clinical settings: access, assessment, diagnosis, treatment, and follow-up. Thus, for example, an ambulatory care visit for severe sore throat might be diagrammed as a core clinical process that includes the following discrete steps:

patient calls practice for an appointment; appointment is scheduled; patient checks in with receptionist; medical assistant rooms the patient and obtains chief complaint and vital signs; clinician obtains history, performs targeted examination, and orders a confirmatory laboratory test; patient receives education on home care and treatment plan; patient adheres (or does not adhere) to treatment plan; and practice contacts patient (or vice versa) three days postvisit to assess progress and to plan follow-up care.

This parsing of even a "straightforward" core clinical process will often reveal multiple targets for improvement. We advise teams to analyze and to map their own clinical activities in these terms and then to attach performance measures to each identified component of the core process. Data can be gathered on key upstream measures to determine their specific relationship to measures further downstream.

In addition, teams can use deployment flowcharts to plan and to monitor the implementation process itself.[4] Even simple tests of change often require substantial coordination. Deployment flowcharts identify specific actors and actions at each step in the redesigned clinical process. Constructing this flowchart facilitates communication between all participants and optimizes sequential handoffs (of both information and patient care responsibility) from one team member to the next.

Managing Change

All clinical change occurs in an interpersonal context and is supported or impeded by both the individual motivations and the collective dynamics of a caregiving organization. Even the best conceived improvement plans will falter if these motivations and dynamics are not effectively managed. We have used and modified several change management guidelines on the basis of the work of Kotter,[5] Reinertsen,[6] and others. These guidelines are offered below, with specific links to the CTS case study:

1. **Understand and communicate the cost of the status quo.** The CTS team compared current costs with expected new costs, and these data motivated participants to embrace the new way.

2. **Develop and communicate the specific vision of a better way.** The CTS team articulated and operationalized its vision over sequential meetings, ensuring collective ownership of the new intervention.

3. **Obtain the commitment of those with the power to make the new way legitimate.** CTS team members spoke with all affected surgeons to gain their cooperation.

4. **Make sure that the change agents have the skills to achieve both human and technical objectives and ensure that individuals are supported and recognized for their work.** CTS team members supported and recognized one another and they worked with each surgeon to ensure comfort with the new location and anesthesia.

5. **Anticipate, understand, and manage the resistance to achieve commitment.** The CTS team negotiated with surgical facilities and discussed the change rationale with all affected surgeons.

6. **Align change with the organization's culture.** The organization is working to emphasize high-value clinical care, and the new CTS activity fit with this value theme.

7. **Leave enough organizational "change reserve" to handle unexpected events.** The CTS team avoided biting off more than it could chew during its first change cycle.

8. **Prepare a thorough change-management plan.** The CTS team developed a flowchart, time line, and critical path to clarify all essential steps in the anticipated test of change.

Linking Improvement Work to Meaningful Clinical Outcomes

The Clinical Improvement Worksheet supports development of tests of change in diverse practice settings. In the present chapter we have traveled with one clinical team as it implements and learns from a specific improvement initiative. Patient-oriented outcomes are the driving force for all such initiatives, defining particular targets for improvement and specifying performance measures for ongoing assessment. The next chapter focuses further attention on these outcomes. We expand our description of the Clinical Value Compass, a tool that complements the Improvement Worksheet, and we explore its utility in defining and monitoring outcomes that are most meaningful to both patients and practitioners.

References

1. Batalden P.: Personal communication to Eugene C. Nelson, Atlanta, 1992.
2. Nelson E.C., et al.: Improving Health Care, Part 1: The Clinical Value Compass. *Jt Comm J Qual Improv* 22:243–258, Apr. 1996.
3. Langley G.J., et al.: *The Improvement Guide: A Practical Approach to Enhancing Organizational Performance.* San Francisco: Jossey-Bass Publishers, 1996.
4. Scholtes P.R., Joiner B.L., Streibel B.J.: *The Team Handbook: How to Use Teams to Improve Quality,* 3rd ed. Madison, WI: Oriel Incorporated, 2003.
5. Kotter J.P.: *Leading Change.* Boston: Harvard Business School Press, 1996.
6. Reinertsen J.: Improving clinical quality. Paper presented at the American Group Practice Association Annual Meeting, New Orleans, 1995.

Chapter 4

Measuring Outcomes and Costs: The Clinical Value Compass

Eugene C. Nelson, Julie K. Johnson, Paul B. Batalden, Stephen K. Plume

When you can measure what you are speaking about, and express it in numbers, you know something about it; but when you cannot measure it, when you cannot express it in numbers, your knowledge is of a meager and unsatisfactory kind; it may be the beginning of knowledge, but you have scarcely, in your thoughts, advanced to the stage of Science. —Lord Kelvin[1]

Health care providers are getting a wake-up call. Outcome-based measures of clinical performance (for hospitals, clinics, and even individual physicians) are increasingly transparent to public scrutiny, and the payment structure for clinical services continues a rapid shift toward "value-based" purchasing. The concept of "value" itself, once an abstraction, has been operationalized by private insurers, commercial employers, and now Medicare itself, in "pay for performance" models of reimbursement.[2] Both patients and purchasers seek high quality at low cost and increasingly align themselves with health care providers and health systems that can meet this demand. Clinicians in this new century will need to demonstrate value and to continually improve it to realize full payment for services rendered.

Real improvement and real value in health care depend on a linking of patient priorities and system processes to specific outcome measurements. The Clinical Value Compass, introduced in earlier chapters, provides a conceptual framework that precisely links values of patients and clinicians to the measurable value that health care systems provide. In this chapter we further develop the notion of health care value, and we explore (in two case studies) the utility of the Clinical Value Compass for understanding and monitoring clinical processes and outcomes in a variety of patient care settings. Our aim is to stimulate readers' use and adaptation of this model in their own clinical work.

Health Care Value: The New Paradigm

A new health care paradigm has gained increasing acceptance among patients, practitioners, and other stakeholders in the delivery of clinical services. The motto might be put simply: "Best quality. Lowest cost. No excuses!"[3] The era of value in health care is now upon us, with *value* defined as a relationship between quality received (or provided) and costs incurred in the receipt (or provision) of that quality.[4] This relationship can be formalized in a simple equation:

$$\text{Value} = f \text{ (Quality} \div \text{Costs)}$$

In other words, the value of a clinical service is directly proportional to the quality of that service (or the quality of benefits that arise from that service) and inversely proportional to the costs associated with that same service. Thus, for example, as costs of an intervention go up, the value goes down, even when quality is held constant.

The advantage of this simple formula is that its basic terms are relevant to, and appropriately understood, by all stakeholders in health care relationships, from patients and clinicians to employers and insurers. From the perspective of health care providers and purchasers, the total cost to the system can be conceptualized more precisely as the product of costs per unit volume and volume of unit services provided or received:

$$\text{Total costs to system} = \text{(costs per unit volume)} \times \text{(volume of unit services provided or received)}$$

Thus, in a technical sense, both these terms (*unit cost* and *volume*) appear in the denominator of the value equation. From the patient's perspective, however, volume is almost always "1" (i.e., the patient himself or herself), in which case the "business" form of the equation reduces to the simpler and more intuitive version offered above.

Those who pay for health care, particularly employers and insurers (but also individual patients, who bear a growing proportion of this burden), focus increasingly on value defined in precisely these terms. Those who provide clinical service, from individual practitioners to regional hospital networks, recognize both the ethical and the financial imperative to concentrate similarly on value-based care.

There is skepticism in some quarters about whether quality and value can be accurately quantified in real-world clinical settings. Great advances have been made, however, in the measurement of health status, health risk, and patient satisfaction.[5] We believe that measuring quality and outcomes is no longer an insurmountable barrier in the documentation of clinical improvement. On the contrary, such measurement is not only practicable but also essential in continuous improvement work.

Indeed, there is growing evidence that providers can use quantitative improvement methods and principles to systematically enhance outcomes and to cut costs. We are impressed by the accomplishments of individual practitioners and clinical teams throughout the United States and in other countries as well. We have witnessed the following, for example:

- Reduction in one hospital's postsurgical wound infection rates from 1.8% to 0.4%, saving the institution $500,000 per year[6]
- Decrease in another hospital's adverse drug reaction rate from 5.0% to 0.2%, saving this institution $450,000 per year[7]
- A 26% decline in northern New England's mortality rate for coronary artery bypass graft (CABG) surgery, representing 82 fewer patient deaths at participating sites[8]

Wise application of continual improvement methods can generate better value in health care settings, just as it has enhanced quality and reduced costs in other sectors of the economy.[9] As discussed next, the Clinical Value Compass integrates components of quality and value that all stakeholders can recognize as important, and it thus empowers practicing clinicians to develop and to sustain meaningful improvements in a wide variety of patient care contexts.

The Clinical Value Compass Approach

We base our discussion of health care value on a series of assumptions that are shared by most patients, clinicians, and payers of health services. These assumptions include the following general principles:

- The aim of health care is to prevent, to diagnose, and to treat disease, and thereby to reduce or limit the burden of illness through restoration, maintenance, or improvement of health functioning.[10–12]
- Health is experienced simultaneously in biological, psychological, functional, and social dimensions.[13]
- Quality health care provides the services (that is, clinical care processes) that are most likely to achieve desired health outcomes at a price that represents value for the patient.[4]
- The value of health care is a function of both quality and costs (per unit volume of service provided or received).[4,14]

How can we pull these assumptions together into a useful, understandable whole? Many models have been applied, but we find particular utility in the value compass approach. As introduced in Chapters 1 and 3 and depicted again in Figure 4-1 (page 49), this approach honors multiple components of patient-defined value and recognizes shifts in these values over time. At the conceptual center of the value compass are individuals or populations who, at a specific point in time, experience a new or continuing health care need: a middle-aged man requires acute management of myocardial infarction; an elderly woman seeks treatment for recurrent depression; parents desire routine immunization for their young child, as part of routine preventive care. These patients can be described at baseline—before a treatment episode begins—in terms of their clinical (biological) status, functional health and risk status, and expectations (what they hope health care can accomplish for them in terms of pain relief, symptom reduction, freedom from physical and mental limitations, and so forth). The patients can also be characterized by the health-related costs incurred over time for management of each particular need. These costs include both direct expenses for medical care and indirect social expenses (including time lost from work) that arise from management of the illness burden. In an important sense, the cost meter for each individual starts running at birth and continues rising until death, taking a jump with each episode of new health need.

As just suggested and reiterated throughout this book, the Clinical Value Compass framework can be applied to people (patients or populations) with diverse health care needs. These needs can be *preventive* in nature, for reduction of future health risk, or can focus on *acute* care of a major or minor clinical problem. Alternatively, ongoing attention might be required for *chronic* care of a single disease or multiple conditions, or for *palliative* care in the context of a life-threatening illness or injury. Most individuals, at different times in their lives, will require all four types of care—preventive, acute, chronic, and palliative—and the health system must be organized to optimize service in all these domains. The Clinical Value Compass framework, in turn, can be tailored to characterize health status and health outcomes in each of these contexts, as they evolve over time in patients' lives. Therefore, the current book includes diverse case studies that reflect the diversity of patients' health care needs and practitioners' care-giving experiences.

The Clinical Value Compass in Figure 4-1 (below) also illustrates the flow of the health care delivery process: the patient accessing the system, then caregivers assessing, diagnosing, treating, and following up with the patient in need. These process steps create a result for each patient or population that can be measured in terms of specific quality-related outcomes and costs. Once again, the patient (or population) can be described after treatment with respect to these same parameters of clinical status, functional status, and satisfaction against fundamental need and pretreatment expectations; and again, this description also includes accumulation of direct and indirect costs during the new treatment episode. As described in Chapter 3, these outcomes are in fact transitions in quality-related health status (clinical condition, function, satisfaction) and incremental costs associated with treatment over time.

We call the circular display of measures—depicted twice in Figure 4-1 (pre-episode and postepisode)—the "Clinical Value Compass," because the layout resembles an old-fashioned, directional compass used for navigation. It has four cardinal points:

- North: functional health status, risk status, and well-being
- East: expectation of health outcomes (pre-episode) and satisfaction with health care and perceived health benefit (postepisode)
- South: costs, both direct (for example, health care costs for physicians, hospitals, drugs) and indirect (for

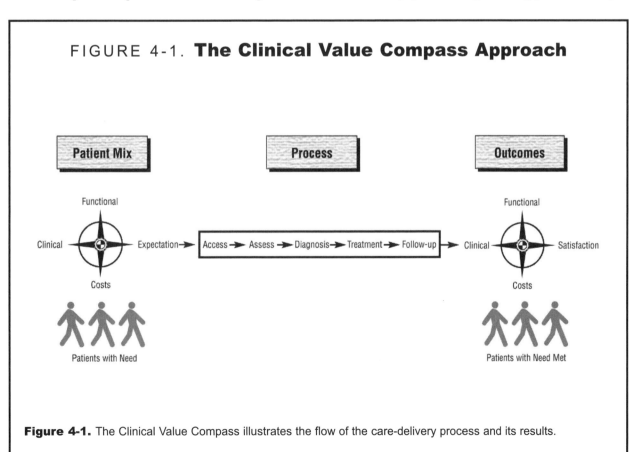

FIGURE 4-1. **The Clinical Value Compass Approach**

Figure 4-1. The Clinical Value Compass illustrates the flow of the care-delivery process and its results.

example, social costs incurred by the family, employer, community)

- West: clinical or biological outcomes (for example, mortality, morbidity, complications)

All four value compass points are important—each in its own right, and because together they circumscribe a balanced and meaningful profile of caregiving outcomes. The territory in each direction can be more or less fully explored, documented, and mapped.

Of course, this heuristic model only begins to capture the rich complexity of patient experiences and clinical services in real-world settings. A truly comprehensive assessment of quality and value would map multiple dimensions of health system structure (facilities, equipment, supplies, personnel) and process (safety, appropriateness, availability, continuity, effectiveness, efficacy, respect, timeliness) against various outcomes of clinical relevance (biological function, mental health, social/occupational capacity, health risk status, health related quality of life), and would extend this mapping to all particular health concerns that might arise in a patient's life (low back pain, depression, chemical dependency, pregnancy and childbirth, and so on). But such an assessment would be costly and prohibitively complex. The Clinical Value Compass simplifies this process, inviting practitioners to select critical indicators of process and outcome known to be important to specific patient populations, and to focus attention on improvement in these domains over time.

Clinical Value Compass Worksheet

As discussed in greater detail in Chapter 3, practitioners who wish to manage and to improve the value of their clinical services will benefit from participation in the following cycle of reflective work:

- Measuring the value of care in specific patient populations
- Analyzing the internal delivery processes that contribute significantly to current levels of measured outcomes and costs
- Running tests of changed delivery processes
- Determining if these changes lead to better outcomes and lower costs

The Clinical Value Compass Worksheet, presented in Figures 4-2 (Side A, below) and 4-3 (Side B, page 51), aids

FIGURE 4-2. **Clinical Value Compass Worksheet, Side A**

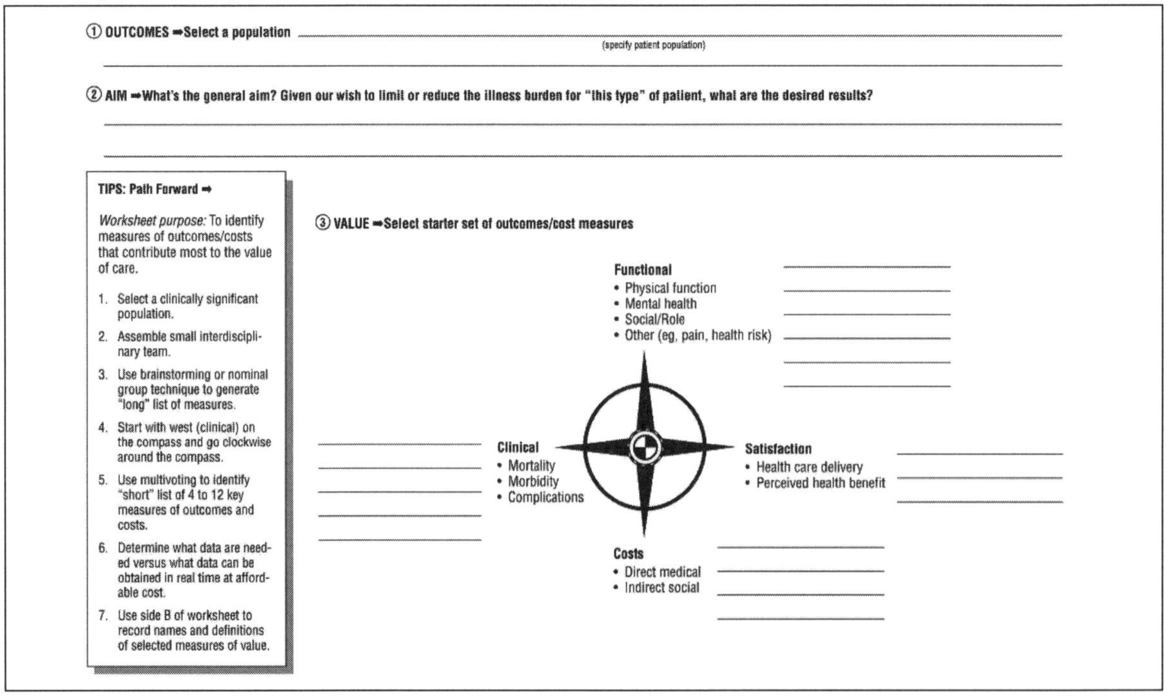

Figure 4-2. Side A of the Clinical Value Compass Worksheet records the identified measures of outcomes and costs. Copyright 1995, Dartmouth-Hitchcock Clinic.

FIGURE 4-3. **Clinical Value Compass Worksheet, Side B**

④ SPECIFIC OPERATIONAL DEFINITIONS ➡ for key outcome and cost measures

TIPS: Writing Definitions ➡

A *conceptual definition* is a brief statement describing a variable of interest. It should tell people <u>what</u> you want to measure and who "owns" it.

An *operational definition* is a clearly specified <u>method</u> for reliably sorting, classifying, or measuring a variable. It should be written as an instruction set, or protocol, that would enable two different people to measure the variable by using the same process and thereby producing the same result. It should explain to people <u>how</u> a variable should be measured.

Variable name and brief *conceptual* definition	Source of data and *operational* definition
A. Owner: _____	
B. Owner: _____	
C. Owner: _____	
D. Owner: _____	
E. Owner: _____	
F. Owner: _____	
G. Owner: _____	
H. Owner: _____	

Figure 4-3. Side B of the Clinical Value Compass Worksheet records operational definitions of key measures for an improvement project. Copyright 1995, Dartmouth-Hitchcock Clinic.

clinicians in this improvement process. The value compass worksheet helps individuals to efficiently identify key measures of outcome and cost (Side A) and to record operational definitions of those measures that are selected for actual monitoring (Side B). Users will recognize a functional connection to the Clinical Improvement Worksheet described in Chapter 3 and elaborated in Appendix A (pages 135–155). Indeed, the two worksheets were designed for concurrent and mutually supportive use.

The Clinical Value Compass worksheet begins with selection of a clinical population and generation of an outcomes-based aim statement to focus the improvement work. The core of the value compass worksheet is the value compass itself. Its four cardinal points offer prompts or cues for the following categories of measurement to be considered early in the goal-defining process:

- Clinical: mortality and morbidity (such as signs, symptoms, treatment complications, diagnostic tests results, and laboratory determinations of physiologic values)
- Functional: physical function, mental health, social/role function, and other measures of health sta-

tus (such as pain, vitality, and perceived well-being and health risk status)
- Satisfaction: patient and family satisfaction with health care delivery process, patient's perceived health benefit from care received
- Costs: direct medical costs (ambulatory care, inpatient services, medications, and so on) and indirect social costs (for example, days lost from work or normal routine, replacement worker costs, caregiver costs)

Using the blank Clinical Value Compass worksheet in Figures 4-2 and 4-3, together with information developed on Side A of the Clinical Improvement Worksheet (Chapter 3), practitioners can prepare a baseline Clinical Value Compass, map out the clinical process in question, and then construct an outcomes-based Clinical Value Compass for the "test of change" process identified.

These initial steps will facilitate the improvement work:

1. Review (and refine, if necessary) the population and aim identified during work in Chapter 3.

2. Starting with the clinical (west) point on the value compass, brainstorm ideas to generate a list of measures that are pertinent to the specified aim.

3. If working in a group setting, use multivoting or another technique to reduce this list to 4 to 12 key outcome measures.

4. Think about what data will be needed, with attention to information that can be reasonably (and affordably) obtained in real time.

The Clinical Value Compass worksheet builds upon Russell Ackoff's advice for problem solvers: "Think up. Think down. Think up again."[15(p. 4)] Ackoff suggests that we first consider the big picture, that we take the long view before homing in on specific facets of a problem to be solved. After working on those specifics and developing a plausible solution, we then reconsider this specific solution in light of larger issues and longer-term aims. In other words, we start with strategy before going to tactics; then we check tactics and actions against strategic intent. This iterative approach is especially useful for facilitators. The value compass worksheet might be most effective when it is not used in a linear manner, straight through from top to bottom. Instead, Side A of the value compass worksheet invites the user to "think up," and Side B to "think down."

When specific outcome variables are selected, they can be further defined both conceptually and operationally. Conceptual target outcomes might include, for example, less pain following surgery, more rapid return to work after an illness episode, or greater satisfaction with the timing of a follow-up appointment. Operationally, these same variables are defined in terms of the method of measurement itself: Who collects the information, and how? Thus, "pain following surgery" becomes "pain score on standardized questionnaire, administered by nurse during follow-up phone call one week after carpal tunnel surgery." All outcome variables must be similarly defined.

How is the Clinical Value Compass approach used to stimulate process improvement and to direct outcome assessment in the real world? We next review two clinical cases in which implementation of the model are beneficial to both patients and health care organizations. We first describe in general terms one ambulatory clinic's value compass–directed improvement of care for women with urinary tract infection. Then we demonstrate the specific application of the Clinical Value Compass worksheet to improve care of patients with acute myocardial infarction in a community hospital.

As emphasized in prior chapters, improving health care is the work of everyone in health care, whether an individual or as a member of a well-coordinated team. The reader will note that our first case below describes clinical improvement initiated by a single general internist in collaboration with her practice nurse; the second case demonstrates collaboration of multiple health care workers in a larger, team-based project. Both models of clinical improvement work are appropriate, and indeed necessary, to optimize quality and value in the varied contexts of real-world clinical care.

Case Example: A Clinical Value Compass for Urinary Tract Infection

Urinary tract infections (UTIs) are experienced commonly by adult women, and the significant discomfort of this condition prompts many individuals to seek care on an urgent basis. A practitioner in a general internal medicine clinic recognized that delivery of such care had not been optimized at her work site, so she invited her practice nurse to join her in an improvement initiative to address specific deficiencies and to enhance value for patients. The physician and nurse interviewed several afflicted individuals and reviewed specific local care processes. They were impressed by experiences like those of Linda, a "typical" patient whose story is shared in Sidebar 4-1 (page 53).

On the basis of this initial exploration, a baseline Clinical Value Compass, Figure 4-4 (page 53) was developed for patients like Linda, and more generally for women in the 18- to 65-year-old age range (the target population for this team's intervention). Similarly, a process diagram was sketched, Figure 4-5 (page 54), depicting Linda's episode of care.

On reviewing these initial data, the clinician and nurse identified several deficiencies in the value of service provided: delayed treatment, multiple urine tests, required office visit with physician, prolonged antibiotic therapy, mandated follow-up appointment, and variable interventions. On the basis of such a process of inefficient care, a post-episode outcomes Clinical Value Compass, Figure 4-6 (page 54), was envisioned.

The physician and nurse reflected on this process and reviewed available clinical literature. After considering several options for tests of change, they decided to implement a nurse-administered telephone-management protocol. They recognized that a small subset of women with UTIs was at relatively high risk for complications and that these cases (which required prompt appointment with a clinician) could usually be anticipated during careful phone screening. Low-risk individuals, however, could be

SIDEBAR 4-1. **Case Example: Uncomplicated Urinary Tract Infection in Women**

Linda, a 40-year-old sales representative, calls her primary care clinic complaining of pain during urination. She has had a urinary tract infection in the past and reports that the symptoms now are the same. The nurse asks her to come to the clinic, but even though Linda is very uncomfortable, she has to make a sales call at 3:30 P.M. and pick up her children at 5:00 P.M. There isn't any way she can visit the clinic before closing time. Linda schedules a clinic visit for first thing the next morning, hoping she won't miss too much work.

Once at the clinic, she waits 90 minutes to see the physician. Linda is a bit upset because she's had to pay for child care for that time and hasn't earned a dime. The physician orders a urinalysis and culture to confirm Linda's infection. Linda leaves with a prescription for antibiotics for seven days and is asked to return for a follow-up urine culture when the prescription is finished. One week later, Linda makes a follow-up visit to the practice, taking more time away from work. The culture is negative.

FIGURE 4-4. **Baseline Clinical Value Compass for Urinary Tract Infection**

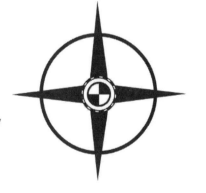

Functional Status
- Pain
- Frequent urination
- Fear of incontinence

Clinical
- Bacterial cystitis
- Urethritis
- Bladder spasm
- Small bladder capacity

Expectations
- Easy access to health care
- Rapid response
- Prompt resolution
- Knowledgeable care

Costs
- Potentially major (if not treated effectively)

Figure 4-4. A baseline Clinical Value Compass for urinary tract infection (UTI) illustrates the clinical outcomes, functional status, costs, and expectations of UTI patients.

FIGURE 4-5. **Original Urinary Tract Infection Treatment Process**

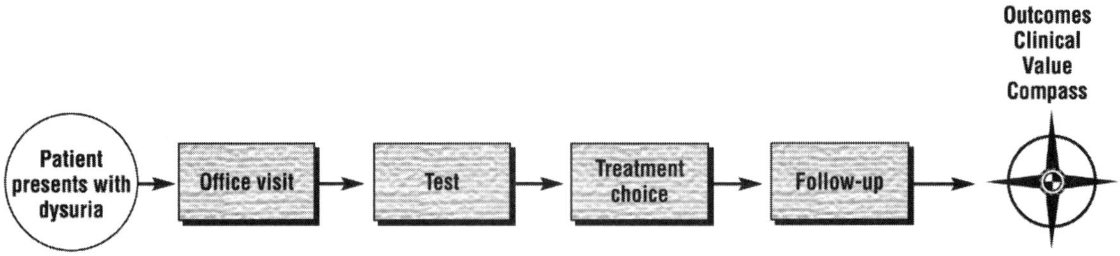

Figure 4-5. The team sketched the original urinary tract infection treatment process, with the results shown in Figure 4-6.

FIGURE 4-6. **Outcomes Clinical Value Compass for Urinary Tract Infection**

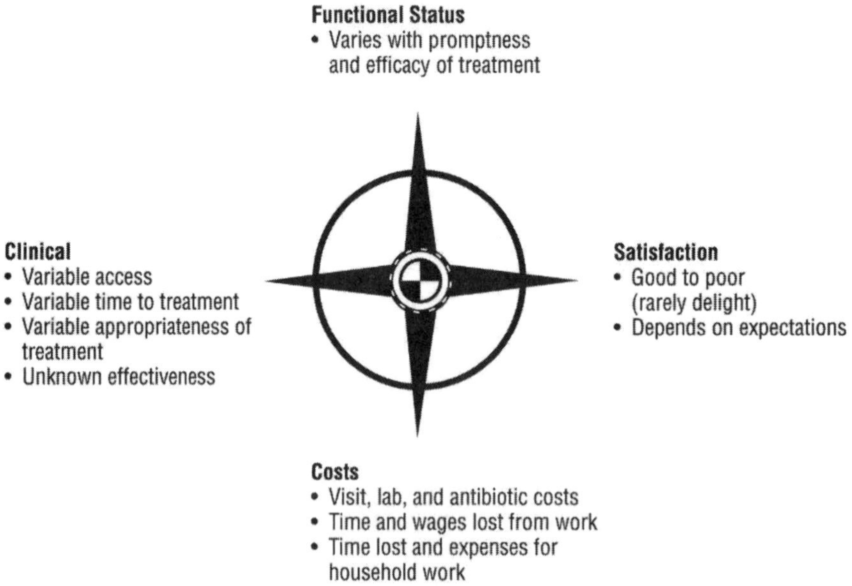

Figure 4-6. An outcomes Clinical Value Compass for urinary tract infection illustrates the variation, high costs, and low satisfaction associated with the original treatment path for urinary tract infection.

served just as well with telephone-based therapy and follow-up. A protocol was thus developed, based on scientifically validated guidelines,[16] to assess specific risk factors via nurse-coordinated telephone screening.

Women at higher risk were promptly and appropriately scheduled for clinician visits. Lower-risk women (as determined by the scripted phone interview) received telephone-based (and protocol-driven) treatment recommendations, prescriptions, and follow-up instructions.

After redesign, the process of care for low-risk patients was considerably smoother and less burdensome for patients, and as shown in Table 4-1 (below), was characterized by fewer unnecessary costs to both the patient and the health care system. Higher-risk women were also

assured prompter clinician attention. As expected, the Clinical Value Compass changed as well, as shown in Figure 4-7 (page 56). The results are clear. The new protocol is effective for screening and treating women at low risk and for appropriately triaging those women whose risk is higher. The patients are happy, even delighted, and the system lowered costs in several areas.

Case Example: A Clinical Value Compass for Acute Myocardial Infarction

Acute myocardial infarction (AMI) remains a leading cause of morbidity and mortality for American adults and a common reason for emergency room presentation and hospital

---

TABLE 4-1. Streamlined Process for Care of Uncomplicated Urinary Tract Infection

Flow of Initial and Revised Process

Initial Process	**Revised Process**
Telephone call from patient	Telephone call from patient
↓	↓
Transfer to appointment secretary	Transfer to nurse
↓	↓
Visit to physician	Structured interview-based history, protocol-driven decision making, data collection
↓	↓
History and physical examination	Telephone prescription
↓	↓
Urine sample for dipstick analysis	Scheduled telephone follow-up
↓	↓
Urine culture	Pharmacy visit
↓	
Prescription	*Time to begin effective therapy: Minutes to hours*
↓	
Pharmacy visit	
↓	
Follow-up visit	
↓	
Follow-up tests	
Time to begin effective therapy: Hours to days	

FIGURE 4-7. **Clinical Value Compass for Redesigned Management of Urinary Tract Infection**

Functional Status
• Prompt return to normal function
• No disruption of work or home life

Clinical
• Prompt clearance for > 95% of patients
• Rare treatment failure
• Rare misdiagnosis

Satisfaction
• 100% delight

Costs
• Antibiotic prescription
• Average telephone time: 8 minutes

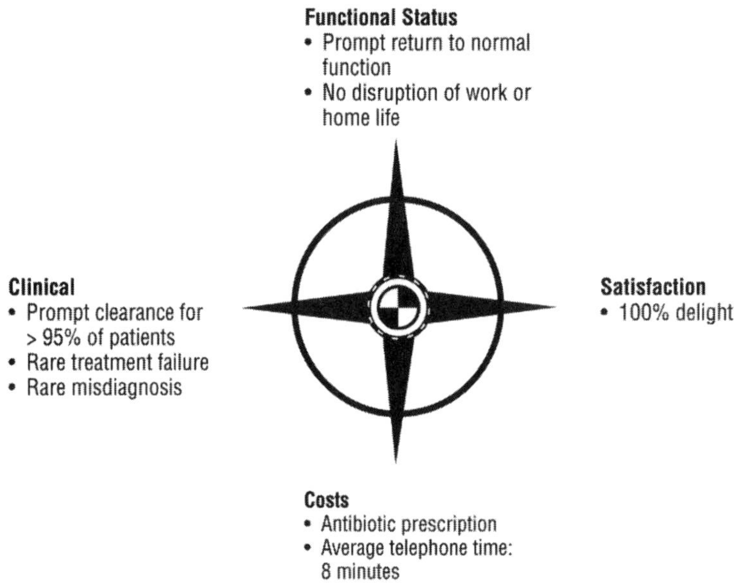

Figure 4-7. The Clinical Value Compass for urinary tract infection (UTI) after the process for managing uncomplicated cases has been redesigned shows the improvements in clinical and functional status, costs, and satisfaction with UTI treatment.

admission. Although timely delivery of evidence-based interventions has been shown to reduce the incidence of adverse outcomes, such interventions are not delivered consistently across all emergency departments and hospitals.[17,18] The Clinical Value Compass worksheet supports exploration and improvement of value-based health care services. Here, we invite the reader to join a clinical improvement team endeavoring to optimize AMI care at a local community hospital. Accompanying figures demonstrate specific use of the value compass worksheet in this case.

Side A—Getting Started: Outcomes and Aim

The process begins with a statement of aim linked to desired outcomes for a target population. This is an invitation to "think up." The aim statement answers the question, "What are we trying to accomplish?"[19,20] In this case, as shown in Figure 4-8 (page 57), the team selects an AMI population for observation over a certain time period: patients with confirmed AMI who are directly admitted to the hospital (that is, nontransfer patients). The clinical process starts when the patients are admitted to the emergency department and ends eight weeks after they have been discharged.

The team selects a clinical population and time period for which the clinical team has primary responsibility for patient care. Next, the team clarifies its aim and writes down its answer to the questions, "Given our desire to limit or reduce the burden of illness for AMI patients, what are the desired results? What's the aim?" The team describes its aim: to find ways to continually improve the quality and value of care for AMI patients.

Although a general aim statement (as just presented) is usually the best place to start, over time most teams will want to revise and to more precisely specify this aim. The increased specificity results from the following:
• Description of the current clinical care process
• Identification of potential changes that are expected to lead to improvement
• Selection of specific high-leverage changes to test using a PDSA (Plan-Do-Study-Act) cycle

Value Measures: Select a Set of Outcome Measures

When designing a value compass, the clinical team can envision important measures of outcome and cost by "circling the compass" in clockwise rotation, that is, by beginning

FIGURE 4-8. **AMI Clinical Value Compass Worksheet, Side A**

① **OUTCOMES➡Select a population** *Patients with confirmed acute myocardial infarction (AMI), direct admissions only, from time of admission to emergency department to 8 weeks post discharge.*
(specify patient population)

② **AIM➡What's the general aim? Given our wish to limit or reduce the illness burden for "this type" of patient, what are the desired results?**
We aim to find ways to continually improve the quality and value of care for AMI patients.

TIPS: Path Forward ➡

Worksheet purpose: To identify measures of outcomes/costs that contribute most to the value of care.

1. Select a clinically significant population.
2. Assemble small interdisciplinary team.
3. Use brainstorming or nominal group technique to generate "long" list of measures.
4. Start with west (clinical) on the compass and go clockwise around the compass.
5. Use multivoting to identify "short" list of 4 to 12 key measures of outcomes and costs.
6. Determine what data are needed versus what data can be obtained in real time at affordable cost.
7. Use side B of worksheet to record names and definitions of selected measures of value.

③ **VALUE➡Select starter set of outcomes/cost measures**

Functional
- Physical function
- Mental health
- Social/Role
- Other (eg, pain, health risk)

Physical function
Overall health status

Death
Angina

Clinical
- Mortality
- Morbidity
- Complications

Satisfaction
- Health care delivery
- Perceived health benefit

Patient satisfaction with hospital
Change in overall health

Costs
- Direct medical
- Indirect social

Total hospital charges
Length of stay
Days lost from work/routine

Figure 4-8. An example of a completed Side A of the Clinical Value Compass Worksheet is shown for patients with acute myocardial infarction (AMI).

with clinical status and proceeding to functional status, satisfaction, and costs. Subcategories of measures are bulleted under each of the Clinical Value Compass axes, reminding users of the types of variables that might be considered under each broad area. Knowledge of the appropriate clinical literature is essential, though its utility is greatly facilitated by complementary knowledge of daily experiences in local patient care. Different team members might bring expertise in different domains. Considered in combination, this diverse base of knowledge and experience will yield a large number of potential measures. Decision-making skills—such as brainstorming to generate ideas and multivoting to reduce the long list to a manageable number of measures—can be very helpful as well.[21]

Note that the Clinical Value Compass worksheet begins with questions that aim to capture clinical professionals' ethical values. Given our desire to limit or to reduce the illness burden for this type of patient, what are the desired results? What's the aim? The patient remains at the value compass's center and focuses our work explicitly on the ethical canon of the healing professions—our ongoing search for better ways to improve patient care.

A word of caution: Although the list of potential outcome measures can be very long, we advise value compass worksheet users to focus initial efforts on a relatively small number of key measures, so that reasonably accurate information can be collected at an affordable cost. Remember, our intention is to improve our ability to characterize the results of care from the perspective of value. As a rule of thumb, 4 to 12 carefully chosen outcome measures are sufficient to get started. Because we often lack any systematically available measures for clinicians' performance, a "developmental" approach to measurement is appropriate. Begin data collection on a small scale: More measures can be added as time passes, as experience is gained, and as information requirements evolve.

This list summarizes the starter set of measures selected by the team for initial monitoring of all AMI patients:
1. Clinical status
   - Death in hospital or within 8 weeks after discharge
   - Angina symptoms

2. Functional status
   - Physical function
   - Overall health
3. Satisfaction against need
   - Patient satisfaction with hospital
   - Change in overall health
4. Costs
   - Total hospital charges
   - Length of stay in hospital
   - Days lost from work or normal routine

The clinical team used nominal group methods and brainstorming to produce a long list of potential measures of outcomes; it then used multivoting to reduce this list to a smaller, more manageable number of measures for which data could be gathered from one of three sources:

1. Medical record review
2. Administrative and billing data
3. Patient-based data gathered by mailed questionnaire (with telephone follow-up of nonrespondents) at eight weeks after discharge

Although the list of outcomes is small, the team did define one or more measures for each of the four value compass quadrants, assuring a "balanced" approach to data collection and quality assessment.

Side B—Operational Definitions of Measures

Side B of the Clinical Value Compass worksheet provides space to record "think down" ideas in the form of specific definitions for key measures of outcome or cost. For each measure, participants create both a conceptual definition (brief description of the dimension or phenomenon of interest) and a precise operational definition (specific, reliable, and understandable process that translates the concept into a reproducible observation on each patient). If the operational definition is based on a previously published or validated measure, the source can be listed on the value compass worksheet as well. Figure 4-9 (below) provides definitions for most of the measures selected by the AMI team. Precision and clarity are essential in the statement of the operational definitions.[22] Reliability and

FIGURE 4-9. **AMI Clinical Value Compass Worksheet, Side B**

④ **SPECIFIC OPERATIONAL DEFINITIONS ➡ for key outcome and cost measures**

TIPS: Writing Definitions ➡

A *conceptual definition* is a brief statement describing a variable of interest. It should tell people what you want to measure and who "owns" it.

An *operational definition* is a clearly specified method for reliably sorting, classifying, or measuring a variable. It should be written as an instruction set, or protocol, that would enable two different people to measure the variable by using the same process and thereby producing the same result. It should explain to people how a variable should be measured.

Variable name and brief *conceptual* definition	Source of data and *operational* definition
A. *Death:* patient dies during hospital stay or within 8 weeks postdischarge. Owner: ________	*Medical record* review indicates patient died, or *follow-up* by mail/telephone at 8 weeks indicates patient died.
B. *Angina:* angina pectoris—pain in chest associated with coronary artery disease (Rose scale). Owner: ________	*Patient's* answers to four questions at 8 weeks coded to form scale: 27. Do you ever have any pain or discomfort in your chest? ❑ Yes ❑ No 28. If no, do you ever have any pressure or heaviness in your chest? ❑ Yes ❑ No 36. Do you have this pain, discomfort, pressure, or heaviness when you walk uphill or hurry? ❑ Yes ❑ No 37. Do you have these symptoms at an ordinary pace on level ground? ❑ Yes ❑ No
C. *Physical function:* the ability to perform physical activities associated with normal living (COOP scale). Owner: ________	*Patient's* answer to one question at 8 weeks: 26. During the past 2 weeks, what was the most strenuous level of physical activity you could do for at least 2 minutes? ❑ Very heavy, eg.______ ❑ Heavy, eg.______ ❑ Moderate, eg.______ ❑ Light, eg.______ ❑ Very light, eg.______
D. *Overall health:* patient's general perception of his/her health status (COOP scale). Owner: ________	*Patient's* answer to one question at 8 weeks: 1. During the past 2 weeks, how would you rate your overall physical health and emotional condition? ❑ Excellent ❑ Very good ❑ Good ❑ Fair ❑ Poor
E. *Patient satisfaction with hospital:* patient's overall rating of inpatient care and services (HQT item). Owner: ________	*Patient's* answer to one question at 8 weeks: 33. How likely would you be to return to this hospital if you ever needed to be hospitalized again? ❑ I'm 100% sure that I'd return. ❑ I probably would not return. ❑ It's very likely that I'd return. ❑ It's very unlikely that I'd return. ❑ I probably would return. ❑ I'm 100% sure that I would not return. ❑ I'm not sure if I would return. ❑ Does not apply to me because I do not live near hospital.
F. *Change in overall health:* patient's perception of the health benefit received from care. Owner: ________	*Patient's* answer to one question at 8 weeks: 7. Overall, is your health better or worse than you expected it to be at this point? ❑ Much better than I expected ❑ Somewhat worse than I expected ❑ Somewhat better than I expected ❑ Much worse than I expected ❑ About what I expected
G. *Total hospital charges:* the sum of all inpatient charges to the patient for the stay, excluding physician charges. Owner: ________	Search of hospital's *billing records* to determine total sum of charges billed to the patient's account for the hospital stay.
H. *Length of stay:* number of days patient stayed in hospital. Owner: ________	*Medical record* review used to determine date of admission and date of discharge; length of stay computed based on interval.

Figure 4-9. An example of a completed Side B of the Clinical Value Compass Worksheet is shown for patients with acute myocardial infarction (AMI).

validity of measures are critically dependent on clear and consistent application of these definitions. The measures themselves will be extracted from data in the medical record, administrative and financial records, and patient reports and ratings at eight weeks after discharge.

When plans for specific Clinical Value Compass measures have been clarified and recorded on the value compass worksheet, the next steps involve designing the following:

- A data collection plan (consider using a simple chart or illustration that describes who, what, where, when, and how for each measure)
- An analysis plan to answer important questions
- A method to display information and to distribute results
- Use of the results for managing patients and improving care[23]

Displays might include graphic depictions of both summary information (for example, results for the first 50 patients) and comparative information (results for this quarter versus a previous quarter; or results of this organization versus another organization). Control charts might be used for individual outcomes or costs, revealing variations and trends over time (a control chart showing length of stay for the past 24 months). A trial or "dummy display"

of measures can be very helpful. The clinical process instrument panel in Figure 4-10 (below) connects process measurements to discrete steps in the delivery of AMI care. Value compass–based outcome results for the project are summarized in Figure 4-11 (page 60).

Advice on the Worksheet Approach

We have used the Clinical Value Compass approach and the Clinical Improvement Worksheet for more than a decade, and we offer these suggestions for their combined use.

Be Flexible. The overall aim is to accelerate clinical improvement, not to slavishly follow any one method for making these improvements. There are two flaws to avoid when making improvements: going too fast (Ready, fire, aim!) or going too slow (Ready...? Ready...? Are we sure we're ready?).

Individual clinicians and larger clinical teams might sometimes benefit from proceeding quickly through Side A of the Clinical Value Compass worksheet and from skipping the construction of precise definitions (Side B) until a specific test of change has been selected. Often, in the case of team-based work, the very occasion of coming together to discuss a common patient care problem will

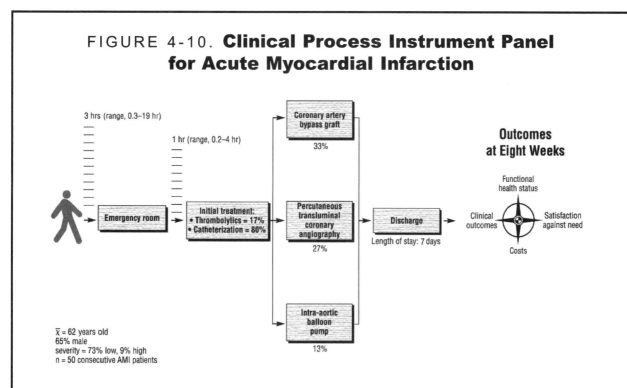

FIGURE 4-10. **Clinical Process Instrument Panel for Acute Myocardial Infarction**

Figure 4-10. The clinical process instrument panel depicts the clinical process for acute myocardial infarction (AMI) care.

FIGURE 4-11. **Acute Myocardial Infarction Outcomes at Eight Weeks**

Functional Health Status
• Overall health: 12% fair/poor
• Patient health rating past two weeks: 70
• Mean time to return to work or routine:
  4.12 weeks

Clinical Outcomes
• Mortality: 16%
• Angina: 16% severe

Satisfaction Against Need
• Overall hospital satisfaction: 83%
• Would return to hospital: 56%
• Communication of clinical information,
  % fair/poor
  — meaning of diagnosis: 18%
  — understanding treatment: 19%
  — knowledge of side effects: 34%

Costs
• Hospital charges: $39,000
• Readmissions: 7%

Figure 4-11. An outcomes Clinical Value Compass for acute myocardial infarction shows the results of the team's work to improve care.

yield many different ideas for improvement. In these situations, there can be value in performing a test of change that all participants agree is worthwhile, even if they do not agree on its relative priority. We often underestimate how much we can learn from the manner in which the system "pushes back" when we try to change it. Making improvements is more important than arguing about which improvement should be attempted first.

When a test of change has been selected by an individual practitioner or agreed on by an improvement team, operational definitions can be created for key outcome measures specific to this intervention. These measures can then be tracked in real time at an affordable cost. If a clinician or clinical group is committed to long-term improvement and repeated tests of change, then a value compass–based data set can be wisely developed that gathers and analyzes information continuously, permitting clinicians to spot favorable trends, to monitor progress, and to quickly detect adverse events.

Start Small. The Clinical Value Compass approach reminds us that quality and value are multidimensional. Practitioners might feel overwhelmed by the large number of potential variables and might therefore feel tempted to

measure everything from the start. This is generally a mistake. The wiser initial strategy is to select a small, balanced set of important outcome measures, chosen because they can be measured reasonably well and because they "hit" each of the four Clinical Value Compass quadrants. New and better measures can be added at any point in the future.

Build Measurement into the Delivery Process. Measurement systems that quantify the quality of patient care are too frequently added on to routine care delivery after the fact. Although this approach permits customized design and standardization, it also adds new costs (in terms of time, labor, and material resources) and thus might reduce actual value. To enhance efficiency and effectiveness, measurement should be built into the care delivery process itself. Frontline providers are thus engaged in both management of the patient and measurement of processes and related outcomes. The new measures can be used in real time to improve care for the individual patient, and they can be immediately accessed to facilitate redesign of care for future patients.[24] Improvement teams must therefore select measures that can be implemented by those involved in service provision itself and that drive the desired quality characteristic of the result.

Clinicians can build measurement into the care delivery process without disrupting care or intruding upon patients. As an example, primary care physicians in the Dartmouth Primary Care Cooperative Research Network and other practices across the United States have built standardized assessment of elderly patients' functional status into the office visit itself, and have found that this assessment not only improves the appropriateness of treatment regimens for the target patient, but also enhances the care of future patients. This is possible because the standardized measures can be aggregated to analyze the functional status of the clinician's entire panel of patients, compared to other similar panels of elderly patients. Point-of-care data collection thus permits generation of a communitywide database.[25] In another example, the cardiac team at Dartmouth-Hitchcock Medical Center has discovered that surgical patients undergoing coronary artery bypass graft have a much higher mortality rate if they must be "returned to pump" during surgery. Therefore, pump clinicians and cardiac team members keep a running count of such patients, monitoring pertinent variables in real time and in aggregate, and use these data in the management of individual patients and collective processes, so that pump returns are minimized.[26]

Use Measurement Instruments Already Available in the Clinical Improvement Literature. Practitioners do not need to reinvent the wheel when devising measurement schemes for parameters of clinical interest. Many simple and validated instruments are publicly or commercially available and can be incorporated into clinical practice with little or no modification. In Appendix C (pages 165–216) we have collected several such instruments, with specific attention to tools that measure outcomes in each of the four Clinical Value Compass domains: clinical status, functional status, patient satisfaction, and cost. We invite the reader to adapt these forms to local caregiving contexts. Further material can be downloaded from a number of useful Web sites, some of which are listed in Appendix E (pages 221–222).

Recognize Limitations. Although the value compass approach enables users to analyze the value of health care and to identify targets for improvement, several limitations must be noted. First, the Clinical Value Compass does not generate prospective information about patient preferences, nor does it identify excess capacity in the system. Second, unless the approach is supplemented by appropriate control charts that document variation over time, important signals cannot be separated from random noise. (See the article by Nugent, et al.[26] for details on construction of Clinical Value Compass–directed control charts.) Third, pursuit of the most rigorous and advanced Clinical Value Compass applications requires mastery of several measurement methodologies (including measurement of clinical outcomes, functional status and well-being, patient satisfaction with care, cost accounting, and financial burden of illness assessment), as well as application of formal analytic techniques (such as summation of rating scales, risk adjustment/stratification, and cost-effectiveness analysis). The availability of validated measurement instruments (such as those provided in Appendix C) simplifies the measurement process somewhat, but does not eliminate the need for sophistication in data collection and analysis.

The logic and utility of the Clinical Value Compass does indeed build on advances in multiple fields of measurement and analysis, and clinician grounding in these various fields can enhance the rigor of application in quality improvement contexts. One strength of the model, however, is that it can be applied with more or less rigor as circumstances permit. Many users have found the Clinical Value Compass framework to be the following:

- Useful in providing a logical and balanced framework for measuring and improving care
- Appealing to diverse stakeholders—doctors, nurses, patients, purchasers, and planners
- Flexible and robust across a variety of caregiving contexts

The Clinical Value Compass can be used in the real world in a more or less sophisticated manner depending on needs, circumstances, available resources, level of experience, and technical knowledge.

Complementary Value Compasses: System Performance

We have emphasized throughout this chapter the utility of value compass thinking to identify patient-oriented outcomes and improvement strategies, but the Clinical Value Compass concept can also be adapted to health care priorities that are less directly clinical. Leaders of health care organizations have used Clinical Value Compass–based instruments to monitor systemwide processes, core operations, and fiscal measures. In Sidebar 4-2 (pages 62–63) we consider a "system performance" Clinical Value Compass that supports strategic planning in small and large health care organizations.

SIDEBAR 4-2.

A System Performance Compass: The Balanced Scorecard

Clinician and nonclinician leaders of health care organizations often use a balanced scorecard of measures to assess systemwide performance in strategic and business domains. This popular approach was developed and refined by Kaplan and Norton[1,2] for use in manufacturing sectors, but it has been widely adopted (and adapted) by service organizations in general (and by health systems in particular) in the United States and around the world.

The balanced scorecard can be effectively depicted in compass format (see figure below) and is animated by four perspectives:

1. **Innovation and Learning.** What must we learn and how must we innovate to be successful in meeting the needs of patients, families, staff, and other beneficiaries? What can we learn from others and from the competitive environment about better ways to meet these needs? What services and products need to be developed, and what processes require innovation?

2. **Core Processes.** What actions and activities need to work efficiently, reliably, and accurately to provide needed services and products? How can we streamline and error-proof our processes? How can we reduce real costs while improving quality, efficiency and beneficiaries' perceptions?

3. **Beneficiaries' Perceptions.** How are we perceived by the (external and internal) beneficiaries of our essential services? How do we compare, in terms of these perceptions, to our direct and indirect competitors? What do beneficiaries expect, want, and need? What delights them and what disappoints them? What prompts defections and what contributes to loyalty? What attracts individuals to our organization and what attracts them to our competitors?

4. **Finance and Growth.** How do our economics look to our shareholders and to our board? Are volumes and revenues growing as planned and needed? Are unnecessary costs being removed without sacrificing technical and service quality? Are we making sufficient margins to build and secure our future? Are human resource assets growing as needed, and where needed, or are we losing human capital in mission critical areas?

Just as the Clinical Value Compass embraces clinical results but extends beyond the biological outcomes into other essential patient-oriented domains, the System Performance ("balanced scorecard") Compass is grounded in fiscal per-

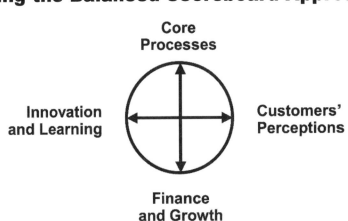

Measuring Organization Performance Using the Balanced Scoreboard Approach*

Core
Processes

Innovation
and Learning

Customers'
Perceptions

Finance
and Growth

* Based on the work of Kaplan and Norton[1,2]

SIDEBAR 4-2. (continued)
A System Performance Compass: The Balanced Scorecard

formance, but extends beyond financial results to incorporate many operational and strategic priorities. In each of these new performance compass domains (innovation and learning, core processes, beneficiary perceptions, and finance), and directly analogous to the Clinical Value Compass itself, users are charged with the following sequential tasks:

1. Define specific objectives.
2. Define measures for each objective and target values.
3. Describe the actions that will be taken to reach the objectives and move the measures.
4. Use the measures to track progress, to make changes as needed, and to use the results for promoting recognition and accountability.

This scorecard compass should be built into annual cycles for planning operations, improvements, and budgets. It is most effective when deployed throughout the organization—from macrosystem to mesosystems to microsystems—and when it engages individual providers as well. For more information on this approach, please refer to relevant articles and books cited in the chapter bibliography.[2]

References
1. Kaplan R.S., Norton D.P.: *The Balanced Scorecard: Translating Strategy into Action.* Boston: Harvard Business School Press, 1996.
2. Kaplan R.S., Norton D.P.: *Strategy Maps: Converting Intangible Assets into Tangible Outcomes.* Boston: Harvard Business School Press, 2004.

Concluding Thoughts: The Value Compass Metaphor—Clear or Confusing?

We have used the value compass as a metaphor to bring to mind four aspects of health care value—clinical status, functional health and risk status, satisfaction, and costs—just as a compass brings to mind four cardinal points—west, north, east, and south. Like the physical compass used for navigation on the open seas or for backcountry orienteering, the conceptual compass of clinical value specifies no inherent hierarchy of its points. All are important. The landscape in all directions is open to exploration, appreciation, and improvement.

But no metaphor is perfect, and some individuals might find the compass image to be confusing. Directional arrows seem to "pull" in opposite directions, and suggest to some users that gains in one territory must be achieved through loss in the several others. Certainly, clinicians are familiar with perceived tensions between high-quality patient care and the economic bottom line or between patient satisfaction and the rigorous demands of disease management. If we consider the interests of other stakeholders, including employers and other health care purchasers, the potential for conflicting "pulls" might be even greater. Providers and patients commonly trade accusations with the organizations that finance clinical care, and compass points become poles at opposite ends of a battleground.

Our own experience, however, is that these very tensions can generate creative solutions beneficial to all stakeholders. The Clinical Value Compass appeals not only to patients and their physicians but also to employers and stakeholders, precisely because it invites a balancing of perspectives and priorities. Cooperation rather than conflict can flourish if all parties gain a deeper appreciation of their common interest in high-value (which equals higher-quality, lower-cost) care. Most stakeholders want patients to enjoy an active, productive, and independent life, and most want to ensure that appropriate clinical care occurs in a satisfying and efficient manner. In addition, controlling unnecessary costs—including health care costs that don't add value—meets the needs of providers, patients, employers, and purchasers.

Our patients, in the end, do not experience themselves as travelers in discrete quadrants of biological, functional, psychological, and financial reality. They live instead as integrated persons at the junction of these several domains. The circle that draws together these separate elements of the Clinical Value Compass reminds us, as clinical experience confirms, that creative work in one domain almost always connects to and stimulates improvement in several others. Real value in health care is achievable in terms that are common to all stakeholders.

References

1. Lord Kelvin (Sir William Thomson) *"Quotations:" On Measurement.* http://zapatopi.net/kelvin/quotes/ (accessed Jun. 25, 2007).

2. Rosenthal M., et al.: Early experience with pay-for-performance: From concept to practice. *JAMA* 294:1788–1793, Oct. 2005.

3. Personal communication between the author [E.C.N.] and Stephen K. Plume, M.D., President, Lahey Hitchcock Clinic, and Professor, Department of Surgery, Dartmouth Medical School, Lebanon, NH, 1996.

4. Porter M.E., Olmstead-Teisberg E.: *Redefining Health Care: Creating Value-Based Competition on Results.* Boston: Harvard Business School Press, 2006.

5. Institute of Medicine: *Performance Measurement: Accelerating Improvement.* Washington DC: National Academies Press, 2006.

6. Classen D.C., et al.: The timing of prophylactic administration of antibiotics and the risk of surgical wound infection. *N Engl J Med* 326:281–286, Jan. 30, 1992.

7. Personal communication between the author [E.C.N.] and Brent James, M.D., Executive Director, IHC Institute for Health Care Delivery Research, Intermountain Healthcare, Salt Lake City, 1995.

8. O'Connor G.T., et al.: A regional intervention to improve the hospital mortality associated with coronary artery bypass graft surgery. The Northern New England Cardiovascular Disease Study Group. *JAMA* 275:841–846, 877–878, Mar. 20, 1996.

9. Womack J., Jones D., Roos D.: *The Machine That Changed the World.* New York City: Harper Collins, 1991.

10. Dubos R.: *The Mirage of Health.* New York City: Double Day Anchor, 1959.

11. Rice D., Feldman J., White K.: The Current Burden of Illness in the United States. In *Annual Meeting of the Institute of Medicine.* Washington, DC: National Academy Press, 1976.

12. Susser M.: Health as a human right: An epidemiologist's perspective on the public health. *Am J Public Health* 83:418–426, Mar. 1993.

13. World Health Organization (WHO): *Constitution of the World Health Organization.* Geneva: World Health Organization Basic Documents, 1948.

14. Donabedian A.: *The Definition of Quality and Approaches to Its Assessment.* Ann Arbor, Mich.: Health Administration Press, 1980.

15. Ackoff R.: *The Second Industrial Revolution.* Herndon, VA: Alban Institute, 1975.

16. Institute for Clinical Systems Improvement: *Urinary Tract Infection in Women, Uncomplicated (Guideline).* http://www.icsi.org/guidelines_and_more/guidelines__order_sets___protocols/womens_health/urinary_tract_infection/urinary_tract_infection_in_women__uncomplicated_2.html (accessed May 24, 2007).

17. McGlynn E.A., et al.: The quality of health care delivered to adults in the United States. *N Engl J Med* 348:2635–2645, Jun. 26, 2003.

18. Peterson E., et al.: Association between hospital process performance and outcomes among patients with acute coronary syndromes. *JAMA* 295:1912–1920, Apr. 26, 2006.

19. Langley G.J., et al.: *The Improvement Guide: A Practical Approach to Enhancing Organizational Performance.* San Francisco: Jossey-Bass Publishers, 1996.

20. Langley G.J., Nolan K.M., Nolan T.W.: The foundation of improvement. *Quality Progress* 27:81–86, Jun. 1994.

21. Scholtes P.R., Joiner B.L., Streibel B.J.: *The Team Handbook: How to Use Teams to Improve Quality,* 3rd ed. Madison, WI: Oriel Incorporated, 2003.

22. Deming W.E.: *Out of the Crisis.* Cambridge, MA: Massachusetts Institute of Technology Center for Advanced Engineering Study, 1986.

23. Nelson E.C., Batalden P.B.: Patient-based quality measurement systems. *Qual Manag Health Care* 2:18–30, Fall 1993.

24. Nelson E.C., et al.: Microsystems in health care: Part 2. Creating a rich information environment. *Jt Comm J Qual Improv* 29:5–15, Jan. 2003.

25. Nelson E.C., Wasson J.H.: Leading clinical quality improvement. Using patient-based information to rapidly redesign care. *Healthcare Forum Journal* 37:25–29, Jul.–Aug 1994.

26. Nugent W.C., et al.: Designing an instrument panel to monitor and improve coronary artery bypass grafting. *Journal of Clinical Outcomes Management* 1:57–64, Dec. 1994.

LEARNING FROM THE BEST: CLINICAL BENCHMARKING FOR BEST PATIENT CARE

Julie K. Johnson, Christina C. Mahoney, Eugene C. Nelson, Paul B. Batalden, Stephen K. Plume

There is always one best result and one best process for achieving that result…and they can always be improved. —Brian Joiner[1]

Why has benchmarking created such interest in health care? Increased competition, the certain knowledge that similar patients are treated very differently, and better communication about measurable variation in outcomes and costs all compel the committed practitioner to learn what works best and to define goals for improvement on the basis of what is learned.[2] Practice-based learning and improvement require that we not only reflect on clinical and administrative processes internal to our own health care setting but also that we turn our attention to both colleagues and competitors to identify gold standards of practice that can inspire and direct our own work. Clinical benchmarking empowers us to identify and to implement "best practices" that we had not previously considered—nor even thought possible.

In this chapter we introduce a process for clinical benchmarking that facilitates the identification and implementation of best health care practices. The process builds naturally on improvement work initiated in earlier chapters of this book, and we make this connection explicit through modification of the Clinical Value Compass (*see* Chapters 3 and 4) for benchmarking purposes. After reviewing basic benchmarking concepts and exploring the value compass–based approach to comparison of practices across different settings, we present two case studies in which benchmarking techniques have stimulated significant improvements in patient care. As in previous chapters, we invite the reader to consider adaptation of these techniques to improvement work in his or her own context.

The Concept of Benchmarking and Its Use in Health Care

We know that the care we provide can be better. The Institute of Medicine (IOM) has estimated that 44,000 to 98,000 individuals die from medical errors each year and that as many as 2% of hospitalized patients experience major permanent injury or death from the medical care they receive.[3] In addition, compelling evidence suggests that Americans receive only 50% to 60% of recommended interventions for acute, chronic, and preventive care needs.[4] If we hope to achieve the IOM's stated goal of health care that is safe, timely, effective, efficient, equitable, and patient-centered,[5] then we must actively attend to improvement of clinical processes and systems at both local and regional levels.

Benchmarking approaches in health care have been adapted from settings outside of health care, where generally accepted definitions of benchmarking have evolved. The concept itself is derived from the Japanese industrial practice *dantotsu*, which refers to a method for finding the "best of the best"—the best practice that consistently produces best-in-the-world results.[6] This idea has spread rapidly throughout the United States and the industrial world. Xerox Corporation, a recognized leader of business process benchmarking, formally defines *benchmarking* as "the continuous process of measuring products, services, and practices against the company's toughest competitors or those companies known as leaders."[6(p.18)] Benchmarking pioneer Robert Camp simplifies this definition to "finding and implementing best practices."[7(p. 237)]

Often the terms *benchmarking* and *benchmarks* are used casually and even interchangeably. In fact, however, these terms differ in meaning, and clarifying this difference is important. The design of effective improvement strategies depends upon appropriate understanding and combining of the two ideas. Benchmarking is a systematic process of searching to identify best practices, whereas benchmarks are statistical measures of the results of a given practice.[8] When benchmarking is performed without consideration of statistical benchmarks, the specific merits of different practices are not fully evaluated. Conversely, if only benchmarks themselves are assessed, no insight is gained into the actual process identified as best practice. In both industry and health care, advocates of improvement often forge ahead prematurely, armed with benchmarks but lacking an understanding of the underlying processes that produced them.

When benchmarking techniques are used effectively and combined with appropriate analysis of resulting statistical measures, the overall process can stimulate local improvement via several mechanisms.[9] Benchmarking processes brings the following benefits:

- Builds awareness of current local capability versus best known capability anywhere
- Encourages people to move from a position of inertia to positive action
- Fosters very different ways of thinking about the conduct of the care/work
- Creates tension for change

These effects are interdependent. An awareness of performance gaps (between one site and another) challenges reflective practitioners to ask why these gaps exist and how they might be minimized. The appreciation of alternate solutions contributes to the tension for change and motivates professionals to work both individually and collectively to achieve such change.

For some organizations (and in our first case study following), an early step in the benchmarking process is to identify partners to benchmark against. Building such relationships enables participants to compare outcomes while increasing appreciation of underlying processes of care. This approach has limitations, however, including the likelihood that benchmarking partners are themselves not "best of the best" in the area targeted for improvement. In this case, the potential increase in performance will not approach best-achievable levels. Although partnerships can stimulate individuals and organizations to expand their own senses of the possible, truly effective benchmarking requires that practitioners look beyond local comparisons of average, normative, or even best performance, and instead (or in addition) explore evidence-based practices documented in the broader clinical literature. Such an approach is outlined later in this chapter.

Nonclinical dimensions of health care provision—such as billing, payroll, and training—can undoubtedly benefit from benchmarking as well. There is no reason to limit this comparative process to nonclinical areas of other health care facilities; excellent benchmarking partners exist in other industries. More than two thirds of health service revenue streams, however, flow through clinical rather than administrative processes.[10] Given this fact, plus our aim to reduce illness burden and to improve value in patient care, this chapter focuses on the use of benchmarking techniques specifically to improve important clinical processes.

Benchmarking and the Clinical Value Compass

The Clinical Value Compass, as depicted in Figure 5-1, page 65 (and described in detail in Chapter 4), can guide practitioners in the benchmarking process. This is true because the Clinical Value Compass' cardinal points define precisely the domains that matter to patients, providers, and other stakeholders, and that therefore are often most worthy of benchmarking investigation. As discussed in previous chapters, these cardinal Clinical Value Compass points delineate clinical outcomes, functional health status, and patient satisfaction along the upper axes. The lower (southern) pole represents total costs, both direct costs of medical care and indirect costs of lost social and occupational opportunity.[11] Initially, the charges paid by purchasers can serve as an appropriate marker of costs in general. As improvement work progresses, however, the indirect costs must be considered as well, if the goal is to identify new ways to minimize the true economic burden of illness.

Our description of the clinical benchmarking process, as described in the following section, uses the Clinical Value Compass as a starting point. Parallel processes occur between internal analysis of one's own organization (as guided by the Clinical Improvement Worksheet described in Chapter 3) and external assessment of similar organizations (that is, of practice sites that serve similar patient populations). The results of this initial benchmarking work then feed back into the Clinical Improvement Worksheet to stimulate additional ideas for change.

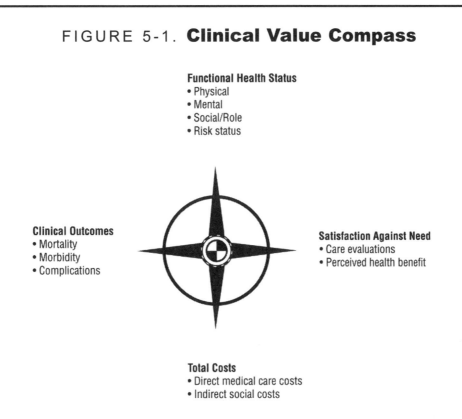

FIGURE 5-1. **Clinical Value Compass**

Functional Health Status
• Physical
• Mental
• Social/Role
• Risk status

Clinical Outcomes
• Mortality
• Morbidity
• Complications

Satisfaction Against Need
• Care evaluations
• Perceived health benefit

Total Costs
• Direct medical care costs
• Indirect social costs

Figure 5-1. The cardinal points of the Clinical Value Compass (west, north, east, and south) show clinical outcomes, functional health status, patient satisfaction, and total costs.

Benchmarking for Best Practices: A Planning Worksheet

A number of models have been described for benchmarking.[12] Motorola uses a five-step process, Florida Power & Light, a seven-step process. AT&T proceeds in nine steps, and Xerox in ten. The distinctions between these several models are not as important as their similarities: All successful processes share several common features. Each reflects a systematic, measured approach to benchmarking that follows a basic format—plan, collect, analyze, and improve.[12] Our own benchmarking model uses this format as well.

A benchmarking worksheet, developed for use with the value compass approach, is shown in Figures 5-2 and 5-3 (pages 68 and 69). Like other instruments presented in this book, the benchmarking worksheet was designed to guide the improvement process, to keep track of results, and to document the work accomplished. Again, the aim of the benchmarking process is to develop testable ideas about best practices. The benchmarking worksheet divides this process into five basic steps:

1. Identify measures.
2. Determine resources needed to find the best of the best.
3. Design the data collection method, and gather data.
4. Measure best against own performance to determine gap.
5. Identify the best practices that produce best-in-class results.

Step 1. Identify Measures

This step defines the statistical measures, or benchmarks, that will focus the external scan (i.e., the search outside one's own setting for best practices). Using the Clinical Value Compass as a guide, users reach consensus on two or three measures for clinical outcomes, functional health status, satisfaction against need, and total costs. Generally, many measures are identified early in the improvement process. During benchmarking work, however, there is value in reducing the number of measures; this will simplify the process of search and comparison, the early part of the benchmarking process. We also recommend that users

FIGURE 5-2. **Benchmarking for Best Practices, Side 1**

Aim: Develop ideas about best practices.

1. Identify measures.
Using the Clinical Value Compass as a guide, reach a consensus on 2 or 3 statistical measures, or benchmarks, that will be the focus of the external scan. Consider the availability of valid comparative data and variability of performance across facilities. (An appropriate benchmark enables measurement and comparison across systems.)

Functional Health Status

Clinical Outcomes

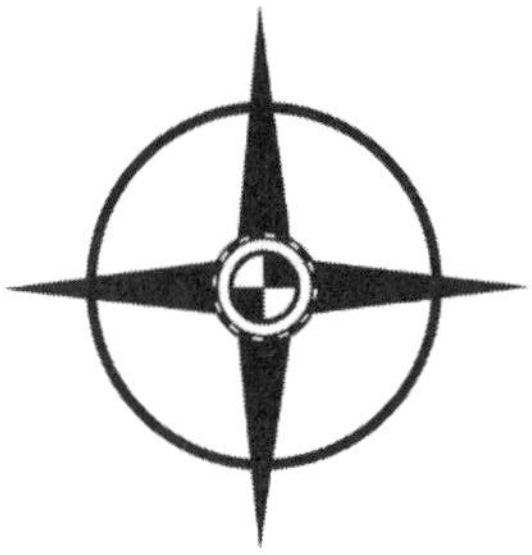

Satisfaction Against Need

Total Costs

2. Determine resources needed to find the best of the best.
Given our desire to limit or reduce the illness burden (cost, resource use, excess morbidity, mortality) for our patients, think about the information needed for finding the best of the best.

The best data to use?
Internal?

External?

The best people to ask?
In-house?

Out-of-house?

The best literature?

Figure 5-2. Side 1 of the benchmarking worksheet helps to develop ideas about best practices by completing secondary research to identify measures and needed resources. Copyright 1995, Dartmouth-Hitchcock Clinic.

FIGURE 5-3. **Benchmarking for Best Practices, Side 2**

3. Design data collection method and gather data.
Who will collect the data? How will the data be analyzed? Who will review the literature?

Task: **Person completing:**   **Date to be completed:**

_____

_____

_____

_____

_____

_____

4. Measure best against own performance to determine gap.
Based on the measures identified in step 1, and the results of an internal and external scan of the data, how does our performance compare to the best of the best?

Summary Data
Number of cases: _____
Total revenue: _____
Revenue rank: _____

Benchmark: _____
Our results _____
Average _____
"Best" _____

Benchmark: _____
Our results _____
Average _____
"Best" _____

Benchmark: _____
Our results _____
Average _____
"Best" _____

Benchmark: _____
Our results _____
Average _____
"Best" _____

Functional Health Status

Clinical Outcomes — Satisfaction Against Need

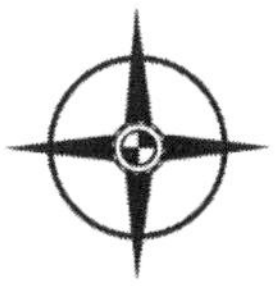

Total Costs

Compared to what we found, how good is our quality and value?

Benchmark: _____
Our results _____
Average _____
"Best" _____

Benchmark: _____
Our results _____
Average _____
"Best" _____

5. Identify the best practices that produce best-in-class results.

Figure 5-3. Side 2 of the benchmarking worksheet organizes data collection and records performance. Copyright 1995, Dartmouth-Hitchcock Clinic.

focus the search on a few key measures from their Clinical Value Compass that have the following characteristics:

- Likely to reflect variability of performance across facilities
- Likely to be available as valid comparison data
- Representative of the important outcomes of care

An appropriate benchmark enables measurement and comparison across locations.

Step 2. Determine Resources Needed to Find the Best of the Best

These resources include the best data, best people, and best literature currently available. Data sources (both internal and external) need to be as accurate as possible to ensure that comparisons are valid and reliable. Internal data might need to be reformatted to allow comparison with external sources. Valuable people resources include in-house experts most familiar with the clinical process, the data, and the benchmarking and improvement processes. In-house experts can usually identify external experts through their professional contacts. The measures identified in the first step can be used as key words to focus the literature search. Most groups benefit from creating a bibliography of those articles that comprise the best literature.

Essentially, this step involves secondary research—querying indirect sources to maximize knowledge on a given subject. In general, the secondary research described here—the best data, people, and literature—won't reveal the actual processes that best-of-the-best clinical sites use to achieve their results. Fortunately, however, providers who offer such benchmark outcomes are usually willing to share their insights into care processes linked to their outcome measures.

Step 3. Design the Data Collection Method and Gather Data

This step establishes a method and time line for data collection and analysis and for review of available literature. The process thus gains focus and is kept on schedule. There is space on the benchmarking worksheet for recording the tasks to be completed, the individuals who will complete them, and the date for completion.

Step 4. Measure Best Against Own Performance to Determine Gap

The team compares best results for each identified measure to analogous measures of its own performance.

Tension for change is generated when a gap is recognized between internal performance and best-practice performance identified during data and literature review. For those benchmarks where comparative data are available, the benchmarking worksheet includes space for internal results, national average results, and the best of the best. To provide interpretive context, space is also provided to record summary data for number of cases, total revenue, and revenue rank.

Step 5. Identify the Best Practices that Produce Best-in-Class Results

At this point, practitioners are prepared to identify processes that produce best results. The work performed thus far supports participants' understanding of relationships between process and outcomes. Tension for change is created, and specific improvement ideas are generated. The organization is now ready to identify potential benchmarking partners and to establish a helpful learning relationship. It is important to optimally understand internal processes and optimally assess external information before potential benchmarking partners are contacted. This knowledge base will make time spent with benchmarking partners more efficient, as detailed understanding will sharpen subsequent questions and improvement interventions.

From Benchmarking to Clinical Care

The work described thus far enables practitioners and larger organizations to clarify their own processes and experiences and to compare these with benchmarking partners or with exemplary practices that have achieved best-of-the-best results. In two case studies, we now explore two different potential next steps in the benchmarking process. First, we briefly examine an explicit benchmarking partnership, the goal of which was to stimulate mutual generation (among participating institutions) of new improvement ideas and higher-quality care. We then present in greater detail the full value compass–based benchmarking process of one regional surgical team that specifically aimed for best-of-the-best practice, and we see how this process stimulated meaningful improvements in patient care.

Case Study: An Example of Benchmarking an Institutional Change Process

Health care organizations can use data from benchmarking work to partner effectively with other sites toward a shared goal of optimizing patient care at all sites. In one illustrative case, several institutions—both academic and community hospitals—began a collaborative initiative to implement rapid response systems (RRSs). The implementation process was rather straightforward, and is illustrated in Figure 5-4 (page 72). The collaborating groups recognized that whereas each RRS would be specifically adapted to its institution, the actual process of implementation was generalizable across institutions.

An analysis of the implementation process across 17 academic hospital sites and 12 community hospital sites revealed key themes that summarized the changes made in practice at each institution. Table 5-1 (below) summarizes key themes for two steps in the Rapid Response Team (RRT) implementation process and provides an example of each theme. These cross-institutional themes and site-specific examples became ideas for what the individual institutions might try in their own setting.

Benchmarking partnerships, such as the RRS collaborative, have the potential to enable participating organizations to share best practices that are at the heart of their own performance, and to learn from best practices performed elsewhere. However, we caution sites to avoid engagement in what Pfeffer and Sutton call "casual" benchmarking, in which well-intentioned efforts fail because organizations approach collaborative learning in a casual instead of systematic way.[11] Casual benchmarking is ineffective because the focus is on copying the most visible and obvious practices, even though these might also be the least important practices.[12] The RRS example illustrates how teams can more systematically explore the means by which their collaborative partners achieve desired results.

In the more extended case study that follows, we walk through a process that is indeed systematic, and we clarify the means by which benchmarking activities can support priorities that patients and institutions identify as most essential.

TABLE 5-1. **Key Themes from the Process Analysis and Examples from Institutions***

Process Step	Key Themes	Examples
Engage Senior Leaders	Senior leaders set RRT as a priority and provided resources	Prioritized by the president as top quality initiative
	Leaders included / assigned to implementation team	Vice president of medical affairs joined RRT work group
	Education provided to • Hospital senior leaders • GME senior leaders • Staff	RRT presentation given to all hospital employees at town hall meeting
	Took opportunities to promote initiative	Posters presented at regional event
	Feedback data to senior Leaders	Report developed for feeding back results to hospital leaders
Provide Education and Training	Education customized for the audience	Hospitalists communicated expectations to moonlighting services
	Developed different methods of education	Telephone stickers with RRT phone number on patient and nursing unit telephones
	Used simulation	Mock RRT events

* RRT, rapid response team; GME, graduate medical education.

Case Study: Using the Benchmarking Worksheet for Improving Bowel Surgery

This example, which is from the Accelerating Clinical Improvement Bowel Surgery Team at Dartmouth-Hitchcock Medical Center (DHMC), highlights key components of benchmarking in real-world practice. Following a general awareness-building session and kick-off event sponsored by the parent institution, an interdisciplinary improvement group was formed to accelerate clinical improvement for patients requiring major small and large bowel procedures in the DHMC delivery system. The five steps defined in the benchmarking worksheet (Figure 5-2, page 68, and Figure 5-3, page 69)—identify measures, determine resources, collect data, measure performance, and identify best practices—were linked specifically with value compass thinking (*see* Chapter 4), and with the Clinical Improvement Worksheet (*see* Chapter 3) to develop an improvement strategy based on process knowledge, benchmarking principles, and outcomes measurement.

The Bowel Surgery Team's completed Clinical Improvement Worksheet (Figure 5-5, page 73, and Figure 5-6, page 74) provides the framework within which this team's work was organized and guides the case discussion that follows.

Team Members → Who Should Work on This Improvement?

The Bowel Surgery Improvement Team included two general surgeons, one senior general surgery resident, one gastroenterologist, one clinical nurse specialist, one enterostomal nurse, one clinical nurse leader, two general surgery clinical administrators, one process consultant, one data specialist, and one team facilitator. They agreed to schedule weekly 55-minute meetings, and they followed structured meeting agendas, designating roles of leader, timekeeper, recorder, and group process facilitator.

① Outcomes → Select a Population (Meeting 1)

The team formed because diagnosis-related groups (DRGs) 148 and 149 (major small and large bowel procedures, with and without complications) represented a large patient population at DHMC with substantial improvement potential. Initial review of external comparative data suggested that DHMC could significantly improve its performance.

What's the General Aim? The team's aim was to decrease the overall average length of stay (ALOS), decrease the mortality rate, increase patient satisfaction, and create the opportunity to better characterize the clinical practices involved in the care of those patients.

Given Our Wish to Limit or Reduce the Illness Burden for This Type of Patient, What Are the Desired Results? The team brainstormed many important possible measures on the Clinical Value Compass:

- Clinical outcomes: mortality, readmissions, success/cure, resumption of diet, and morbidity measures—intra-abdominal, cardiac, and pulmonary complications; wound infection; and additional corrective surgery
- Functional health status: physical and mental health based on the SF-36® or SF-12® health surveys[13]

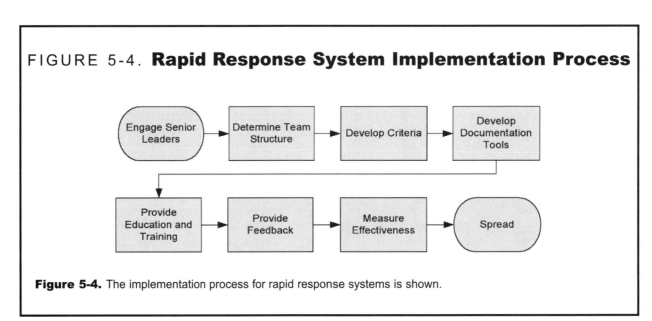

FIGURE 5-4. **Rapid Response System Implementation Process**

Figure 5-4. The implementation process for rapid response systems is shown.

- Satisfaction: patient and family education, registered nurse caring and concern, diet and nutrition, timeliness and access from clinic visit to operation date, ease of transition (from office to hospital, one hour after surgery, hospital to home), congruence of outcomes with expectations

- Costs: direct costs (preoperative, operative, hospital charges, professional [surgical] fees, and visiting nurses) and indirect costs (loss of work, family and child care, and out-of-pocket expenses)

Step 1. Identify Measures

The team reached consensus on a few high-priority benchmarks for each of the Clinical Value Compass points:

- Clinical outcomes: mortality, morbidity, infection rate, and surgical technique

- Functional health status: pain management, physical function, and psychosocial health
- Satisfaction: patient and family satisfaction and patient and family perspective
- Costs: length of stay, total charges, and indirect social costs

Step 2. Determine Resources Needed to Find the Best of the Best

For the best internal data, the group focused on statistical measurement and graphic display of key data points related to the surgical care process. The best sources of external data available to the group were the large administrative databases of the New Hampshire Hospital Association and the Academic Medical Center Consortium. Scanning the internal data suggested areas of process variability amenable to further investigation.

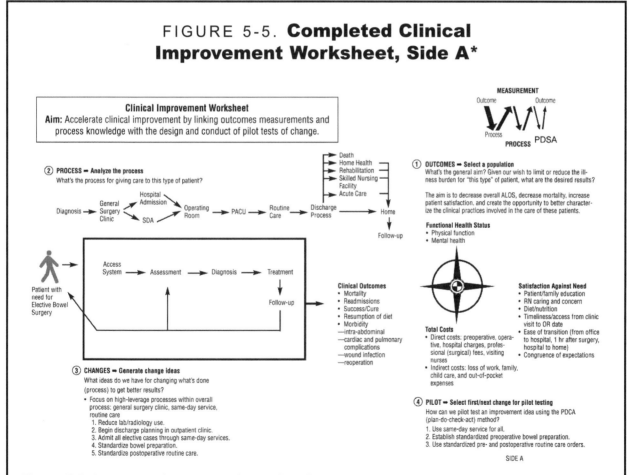

Figure 5-5. An example of a completed Side A of the Clinical Improvement Worksheet is shown for Bowel Surgery Improvement Team. * ALOS, average length of stay; OR, operating room; PACU, postanesthesia care unit; PDSA, Plan-Do-Study-Act (cycle); RN, registered nurse; SDA, same-day service area.

FIGURE 5-6. **Completed Clinical Improvement Worksheet, Side B***

Making Improvements: Clinical Improvement Worksheet

TEAM MEMBERS ➡ **Who should work on this improvement?**

1. _Leader_
2. _Facilitator_
3. _2 surgeons_
4. _1 general surgery resident_
5. _1 process consultant_
6. _1 gastroenterologist_

7. _1 clinical nurse specialist_
8. _1 enterstomal nurse_
9. _1 clinical nurse leader_
10. _2 general surgical clinical administrators_
11. _1 data specialist_

Coach _____   Administrative Support _____

Ⓐ **AIM** ➡ **What are we trying to accomplish? (more specific aim)**

An opportunity exists to improve the surgical care of patients undergoing surgery of the small and large bowel beginning with the diagnosis and ending 30 to 60 days after discharge.

Ⓑ **MEASURES** ➡ **How will we know whether a change is an improvement?**

• Decreased length of stay
• Decreased mortality rate compared with DHMC 1992 data and AMCC data
• Increased patient satisfaction

Ⓒ **SELECTED CHANGE** ➡ **How would you describe the change that you have selected for testing?**

First Cycle:
1. Admit all elective cases through same-day services.
2. Standardize the outpatient bowel preparation process.
3. Develop and implement a standard order set for the first postoperative day.

Second Cycle:
1. Develop a clinical pathway for bowel surgery patients.
2. Implement clinical pathway for the elective surgery population.

Ⓓ **PLAN** ➡ **How shall we** _plan_ **the pilot?**

• Who? Does what? When? With what tools and training?

For the clinical pathway trial, in-service training was provided by the nursing members of the bowel surgery team to the outpatient general surgery staff, the same-day services program, and the two inpatient surgical units. The participating surgeons provided orientation to the General Surgery Section attendings and housestaff. A resource binder was developed to provide housestaff and nursing staff an overview of the pathway and articles which support the clinical content of the pathway's order set.

• Baseline data to be collected?

Length of stay, total charges, charges categorized by medications, laboratory tests, PACU and OR charges, proxies for functional health status, and patient satisfaction.

Ⓔ **DO** ➡ **What are we learning as we** _do_ **the pilot?**

• Shading the physician's order set made it difficult for the pharmacists to read the medication orders.
• The tracking sheet used to identify elective patients scheduled for surgery needed to be optimized so that their progress could be better monitored by a team member.
• Compliance with use of the pathway was higher on the unit where the _team_ member followed the patients each day to answer nursing and housestaff questions and to follow up on incomplete documents.
• The goal of mobilizing the patient immediately after surgery was generally delayed until the first postoperative day.

Ⓕ **STUDY** ➡ **As we** _study_ **what happened, what have we learned?**

• Did original outcomes improve?

Yes, summarized and illustrated in the text.

Ⓖ **ACT** ➡ **As we** _act_ **to hold the gains or abandon our pilot efforts, what needs to be done?**

The team continues to meet on a monthly basis to discuss progress of pathway patients.

Figure 5-6. An example of a completed Side B of the Clinical Improvement Worksheet is shown for the bowel Surgery Improvement Team. * ALOS, average length of stay; OR, operating room; PACU, postanesthesia care unit; PDSA, Plan-Do-Study-Act (cycle); RN, registered nurse; SDA, same-day service area.

DHMC physicians and other experts most familiar with the clinical process were recruited for the analysis. The group discovered that clinical experts (nationally recognized surgical leaders) existed within their own system and were already active participants in the improvement process. Additionally, these internal experts had been networking with their national colleagues for years before initiation of this new improvement effort. The decision was made to delay formal contact with external regional and national experts until later in the improvement process. The group wanted to first develop complete familiarity with current sources of variation within its own system of medical care delivery. Only after establishing such knowledge did the team proceed to the identification of gaps between its own process and the processes used by best-known surgical teams nationwide.

Working with a clinical reference librarian, the benchmarker (that is, the person leading benchmarking efforts for the team) focused on measures identified in Step 1, and searched the available literature using the online databases MEDLINE® and CINAHL®. As the benchmarker scanned search results to identify best articles on bowel surgery, she developed a bibliography that could be shared with group members and easily updated over time.

Step 3. Design the Data Collection Method and Gather Data

Assigned tasks included running internal data reports, constructing graphic displays of the data, periodically updating the literature review, and creating a condition-specific bibliography. The group also set a date for a "state of the union" address and kick-off event, during which results of the benchmarking process would be presented to the entire improvement team. A reunion of all the participating care sites was scheduled for six months after this general launch. The purpose of the reunion was to report on progress made and to share lessons learned with colleagues at multiple DHMC sites who were engaged in similar improvement efforts.

At this point, the group hit a roadblock that many improvement teams experience—the participants became paralyzed by the amount of data available (that is, paralysis by the magnitude of analysis). This volume of data, coupled with discussions of different analysis methods, slowed the team's progress. Delays in data acquisition and formatting also set back the work. This latter issue was partially resolved through setting more realistic expectations about time involved in data analysis. Significant time is required to sort through questions of data validity, formatting, and analysis. As the project progressed, the medical center's information systems made available a reporting tool based on a graphical query language. This allowed individual users to access databases and to display results more effectively as spreadsheets and graphs. This development, in turn, reduced turnaround time involved in data analysis. Finally, the group found that focusing on previously identified Clinical Value Compass measures helped to limit the scope of their data requests and analyses.

Step 4. Measure Best Against Own Performance to Determine Gap

The benchmarker identified specific measures of internal quality and costs that could be compared to the best of the best. Comparable data for functional health status and satisfaction measures were not obtainable, but measures of mortality, length of stay, and total charges were discovered and reviewed. The literature also revealed that gains could be made in pain management.

Step 5. Identify the Best Practices that Produce Best-in-Class Results

The benchmarking results (shown in Figure 5-7, page 76, and Figure 5-8, page 77) revealed a substantial gap between local results and those produced by best-known teams at comparable organizations. When the DHMC group considered these findings, it rapidly reached the following conclusions:

- The data were far from perfectly accurate, so that fair, careful comparisons were difficult to make; nevertheless, the information was still useful for identifying potential improvement areas. The team decided to break out elective cases from urgent cases to clarify the results for each respective stratum.

- Reduction in ALOS was a high-priority improvement opportunity.

- The exact survival rate was not known, but it was possible that a gap existed between the current team's rate and the best survival rate.

- Although hospital charges to payers do not necessarily reflect actual costs of care, a significant difference in charges was noted between DHMC and the provider with the lowest charge. As a result, the team became curious about specific components of DHMC charges.

- Accurate comparative data on functional health status and patient satisfaction were scarce. Unpublished data suggested that some medical centers were doing substantially better, yet none appeared to have reached maximum achievable levels of performance.

- Because the team recognized that benchmarking should be an ongoing process, it continued to assess best practices even after concentration on local improvement strategies.

As the benchmarking work proceeded, the Bowel Surgery Team continued to push forward using the Clinical Improvement Worksheet. Further progress is summarized in the following sections.

② Process → Analyze the Process (Meeting 2)

What's the Process for Giving Care for This Type of Patient? The bowel surgery process was detailed on a flowchart (*see* Figure 5-5 on page 73), beginning with diagnosis and ending 30 to 60 days after discharge (at the first follow-up clinic appointment).

③ Changes → Generate Change Ideas (Meeting 3)

What Ideas Do We Have for Changing What's Done (Process) to Get Better Results? Using the flowchart developed for analysis of surgical care, the team identified high-leverage steps within the overall process: general surgery clinic, same-day service, and routine care. Ideas for changing the general surgery clinic process included reduced use of preoperative laboratory and radiology resources, and initiation of discharge planning at time of preoperative outpatient visit. In the same-day services area, change ideas included admission of all elective cases through same-day services, and standardization of the bowel-preparation procedure. Finally, the team decided

FIGURE 5-7. **Completed Benchmarking Worksheet, Side 1***

Benchmarking for Best Practices

Aim: Develop ideas about best practices.

1. Identify measures.
Using the Clinical Value Compass as a guide, reach a consensus on 2 to 3 statistical measures, or benchmarks, that will be the focus of the external scan. Consider the availability of valid comparative data and variability of performance across facilities. (An appropriate benchmark enables measurement and comparison across systems.)

Physical and

psychosocial health

Pain management

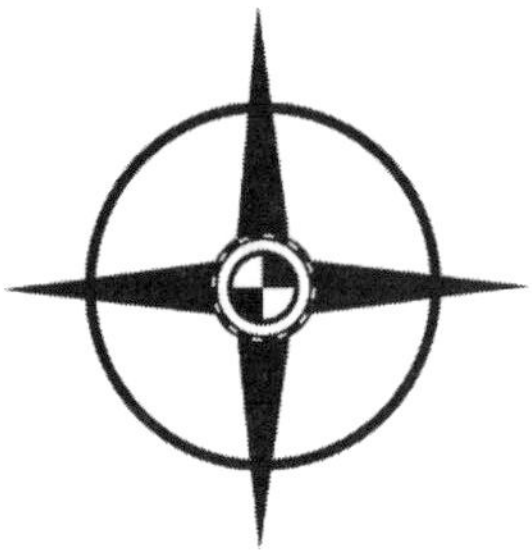

Functional Health Status

Clinical Outcomes

Mortality

Morbidity

Infection rate

Surgical technique

Satisfaction Against Need

Patient/family satisfaction

Patient/family perspective

Total Costs
Length of stay

Total charges

Social costs

2. Determine resources needed to find the best of the best.
Given our desire to limit or reduce the illness burden (cost, resource use, excess morbidity, mortality) for our patients, think about the information needed for finding the best of the best.

The best data to use?
Internal?

- Focus on statistical measurement and graphic display of key data points related to patient care process.

External?

- NHHA Database
- AMCC Database

The best people to ask?
In-house?

- Focus on developing multidisciplinary team.

Out-of-house?

- Identify key clinical experts in the field for future consultation.

The best literature?

- Search the literature using MEDLINE, CINAHL.
- Create electronic bibliographic database.

Figure 5-7. An example of a completed Side 1 of the benchmarking worksheet is shown for the Bowel Surgery Improvement Team. * AMCC, American Medical Center Consortium (now the Association of American Medical Colleges); NHHA, New Hampshire Hospital Association.

FIGURE 5-8. **Completed Benchmarking Worksheet, Side 2***

3. **Design data collection method and gather data.**
   Who will collect the data? How will the data be analyzed? Who will review the literature?

Task:	Person completing:	Date to be completed:
Produce data reports.	A. Hinkle	
Create data displays.	A. Hinkle, B. Swartz	
Search literature.	C. Mahoney	
Create bibliography.	C. Mahoney	

4. **Measure best against own performance to determine gap.**
   Based on the measures identified in step 1, and the results of an internal and external scan of the data, how does our performance compare to the best of the best?

Benchmark: _Pain management_

Our results _Not available_

National Average _Not available_

Best _Not available_

Summary Data	
Number of cases:	170
Total revenue:	> $5 million
Revenue rank:	#8

Benchmark: _Surgical technique_

Our results _Not available_

National Average _Not available_

Best _Not available_

Benchmark: _1993 total hospital charges_

Our results $34,000

National Average $33,000

Best $14,000

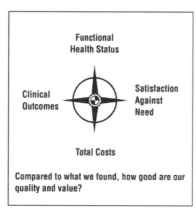

Compared to what we found, how good are our quality and value?

Benchmark: _Patient/family satisfaction_

Our results _Not available_

National Average _Not available_

Best _Not available_

Benchmark: _1993 mortality*_

Our results > 3%

National Average 3%

Best < 1%

*Note: This illustrates the results of an initial benchmarking effort in November 1994, comparing DHMC to other major medical centers. Data have been adjusted for case mix, but include both urgent and elective cases as well as complicated and uncomplicated cases.

Benchmark: _1993 length of stay_

Our results 16

National Average 14

Best 10

5. **Identify the best practices that produce best-in-class results.**

Figure 5-8. An example of a completed Side 2 of the benchmarking worksheet is shown for the Bowel Surgery Improvement Team. * DHMC, Dartmouth-Hitchcock Medical Center.

that standardized orders for postoperative care could promote more appropriate use of medications and laboratory, and could facilitate nasogastric tube management, resumption of feeding and ambulation, and ancillary consultations (for example, physical therapy, occupational therapy).

These changes were incorporated into development of a clinical pathway for this patient population. To address issues of patient satisfaction and functional health status, the team collaborated with an existing internal consulting group to perform routine telephone follow-up surveys. All patients undergoing large and small bowel surgery would be surveyed four weeks after discharge to gather feedback on functional status and satisfaction. In addition, members of the improvement group continued to review potential tools for measurement of health status and satisfaction, and development of a condition-specific survey was also considered.

④ Pilot → Select a Change for Pilot Testing (Meeting 4)

How Can We Pilot Test an Improvement Idea Using the PDSA Method? The team planned three successive PDSA cycles, beginning with the least complex change and progressing toward changes perceived as more difficult. Each test of change moved the process up an "improvement ramp" of increasing complexity, as depicted in Figure 5-9 (page 79). The first three initiatives were implemented, and data related to these steps were collected. These initiatives included the following:

- Using same-day services for all elective surgery patients
- Establishing a standardized preoperative bowel preparation procedure
- Using standard preoperative and postoperative care orders

Results and Lessons Learned

The results were very encouraging. ALOS was reduced from 9.3 days to 5.1 days, readmissions within 30 days decreased by more than 50%, and patient satisfaction improved from 86% to 93%. Overall readmission rates also fell. As the team continued to analyze data and to make further improvements, it used control charts to monitor data over time.

After working through this process, participants discovered that many barriers to implementation had been eliminated. The initial selection of group members was one key to successful implementation. Including the two most senior attending surgeons in the group immediately engaged the clinical staff; these physicians' support decreased resistance among other attending surgeons and house staff. Other participating caregivers were able to anticipate resistance and work out implementation problems. Finally, the team obtained input from other medical specialists and achieved consensus before formalizing its planned changes.

Members of the original Bowel Surgery Team continued their collaborative work and identified several further areas for improvement. Overall and surgeon-specific instrument panels were created to document trends in patient mix, key process variables (for example, operating room hours, postanesthesia care unit hours, operating room charges, counts of medications and laboratory tests), and outcomes- and cost-related variables (mortality, readmissions, functional health status, length of stay, hospital charges). Data comparing surgeons to each other and to the section average were compiled every six months. All surgeons were able to identify themselves but not other surgeons. For several years, reports were used to monitor performance and to further refine care processes over time.

Substantial effort went into subsequent development and implementation of a critical pathway that built straightforward standing orders into the care delivery process. Despite the team's success in implementing earlier changes, and despite efforts to reach consensus and provide education and support, the new standing orders met with significant resistance. Some barriers to acceptance seemed to be cultural, including, for example, concerns about "cookbook medicine." Another issue was appropriate management of patients who "fell off" the pathway. Finally, and notably, the team had decided early in its work to not hold just one person accountable for this new pathway; in retrospect, this lack of a point person and champion might have added to the implementation difficulties.

Even with challenges specific to one of the work group's specific projects, Clinical Value Compass–defined outcomes were tracked for several more years. These data confirmed that improvements in clinical outcomes, cost, and satisfaction persisted over the time frame of active monitoring. Thus, improvements in care were not only achievable, but also (for several subsequent years) sustainable.

Comments and Conclusions

The bowel surgery case illustrates some important points that should be kept in mind as clinicians prepare to use benchmarking techniques to improve local care.

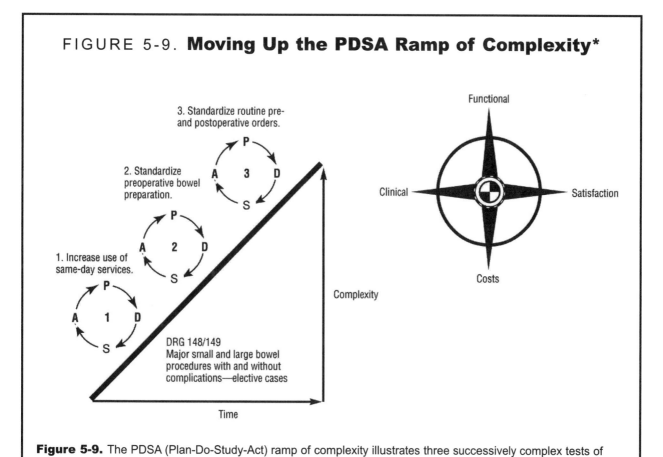

FIGURE 5-9. **Moving Up the PDSA Ramp of Complexity***

Figure 5-9. The PDSA (Plan-Do-Study-Act) ramp of complexity illustrates three successively complex tests of change in bowel surgery care. * DRG, diagnosis-related group.

Someone, Somewhere Is Best. Although it might not be a single provider, someone, somewhere does practice in a way that produces the best results in clinical outcomes, functional status, satisfaction, and costs. Learning about those best practices is the aim of benchmarking.

Even the best are not the ideal. A truly optimal health system must include knowledge about relevant treatment options freely and accurately communicated to patients, decision making on therapeutic actions shared by patients and clinicians, continual improvement of the process of care, continual assessment and reassessment of conventional treatment modalities, and identification and reallocation of excess capacity. Such a system is usually somewhere beyond both one's own current performance and existing best-known practices.

Benchmarking Is (Just) a Tool. Although benchmarking is a useful tool for understanding and learning about current best practices, it is just one step in the journey toward optimal health care delivery.

Benchmarking Creates Tension for Change. Benchmarking goes beyond the mere replication of what others are doing to achieve similar outcomes. Instead, benchmarking can generate the tension for change that leads to innovative performance and breakthrough results.

Benchmarking Is an Ongoing Process. As best practices and best outcomes continue to evolve, benchmarking will help clinicians to continually assess the external environment.

Although we have emphasized throughout this book that clinical improvement is the job of everybody and that this work can be undertaken both by individual practitioners and by loosely or highly organized work groups, the process of benchmarking is especially conducive to collaborative interactions. Effective benchmarking groups combine the clinical experiences of frontline practitioners and staff with the analytic, quantitative, and qualitative skills of data and benchmarking coordinators. Of course, these role boundaries can be highly permeable. Although the leader of benchmarking activities need not be a practicing clinician, this individual will benefit from familiarity with the processes of patient care and from a regular working relationship with the clinical staff. Indeed, Camp and Tweet emphasize the importance of all team members being actively involved in the work of their own benchmarking: "When the process owners conduct their own benchmarking, they develop a commitment to the process and the resulting best practices."[7(p. 237)] Finally, both concerted management support and carefully designed communication are essential for all effective benchmarking processes.[13]

In a health care environment that has grown increasingly transparent to patients, purchasers, and other clinical providers, with quality and cost data more available for public scrutiny, and with improvement collaboratives more frequently utilized for shared learning, benchmarking knowledge and benchmark data are increasingly easy to obtain. Appropriate use of comparative measurements can stimulate wise clinical changes and demonstrable improvements in quality and value. Benchmarking locates these improvements in the context of the rest of the known world. Moving into the rest of that world is an important aspect of the work in the next several chapters, which reconsider the process of change in both individuals and institutions.

References

1. Joiner B.: Reflections on Dr. Deming's contributions to management. Closing keynote address at the Eighth Annual International Deming User's Group Conference. Ohio Quality and Productivity Forum, Cincinnati, Aug. 17, 1994.
2. Wennberg J.H., et al.: *The Dartmouth Atlas of Health Care: 1996.* Chicago: American Hospital Publishing, 1996.
3. Institute of Medicine: *To Err Is Human: Building a Safer Health System.* Washington, DC: National Academy Press, 2000.
4. McGlynn E.A., et al.: The quality of health care delivered to adults in the United States. *N Engl J Med* 348:2635–2645, Jun. 26, 2003.
5. Institute of Medicine: *Crossing the Quality Chasm: A New Health System for the 21st Century.* Washington, DC: National Academy Press, 2001.
6. Camp R.C.: *Business Process Benchmarking: Finding and Implementing Best Practices.* Milwaukee: ASQC Quality Press, 1995.
7. Camp R.C., Tweet A.G.: Benchmarking applied to health care. *Jt Comm J Qual Improv* 20:229–238, May 1994.
8. Bogan C.E., English M.J.: *Benchmarking the Best Practices: Winning Through Innovative Adaptation.* New York City: McGraw-Hill, 1994.
9. Mosel D., Gift B.: Collaborative benchmarking in health care. *Jt Comm J Qual Improv* 20:239–249, May 1994.
10. Campbell B.: Benchmarking: A performance intervention tool. *Jt Comm J Qual Improv* 20:225–228, May 1994.
11. Pfeffer J., Sutton R.: *Hard Facts: Dangerous Half-Truths & Total Nonsense.* Boston: Harvard Business School Press, 2006.
12. American Productivity & Quality Center: *The Benchmarking Management Guide.* Cambridge, MA: Productivity Press, 1993.
13. Ware J.E. Jr., et al.: *The MOS SF-36 Health Survey and the MOS SF-12 Health Survey.* Boston: The Health Institute, New England Medical Center, 1995.

BUILDING ON CHANGE: CONCEPTS FOR IMPROVING ANY CLINICAL PROCESS

Paul B. Batalden, Julie K. Johnson, Eugene C. Nelson, Stephen K. Plume, Joel S. Lazar

Until you can see a different reality, you are hard-pressed to do anything differently. —John Kelsch[1]

As young practitioners achieve mature professional competence, they approach clinical pattern recognition and problem solving with increasingly reflective and integrative forms of reasoning. In a recursive and largely spontaneous process that Donald Schön refers to as "reflection-in-action,"[2] seasoned professionals combine inquiry, intervention, and evaluation to generate higher-order conceptions of complex clinical realities. Where novice clinicians register isolated details of history and physical exams and apply formal algorithms to solve standard problems, experienced practitioners combine technical facility with intuitive appreciation, and derive elegant therapeutic strategies that are both creative and clinically sound.

Earlier chapters introduced practice-based learning and improvement with a similar developmental trajectory in mind. The work of quality innovation is well supported by tools such as the Clinical Improvement Worksheet (Chapter 3) and the Clinical Value Compass (Chapter 4), but experienced practitioners of improvement will appreciate the extent to which such instruments are means rather than ends in the important work of enhancing health care value. With growing experience, clinicians' initially algorithmic view of systemwide patterns and processes grows increasingly reflective and intuitive. Improvement solutions become increasingly generalizable in their structure, though no less specific in their implementation.

In the current chapter, and in Chapters 7 through 9, we cycle back on issues explored in previous chapters of this book, but (as in the iterative process of Plan-Do-Study-Act, [PDSA] cycles themselves) we explore these issues from a perspective of greater experience, and we recognize solutions of broader scope.

Can we, for example, reconsider Chapter 2's "Strategies to Target Clinical Care and Costs," and now think more broadly about both stimuli and barriers to change? The current chapter explores underlying *change concepts* that support the generation and elaboration of specific improvement ideas. We walk the reader through an illustrative case study in which change-concept thinking both broadens and deepens clinicians' understanding of improvement possibilities. Readers are invited to reflect on their own guided improvement experiences in previous chapters and to draw higher-level connections between past and future opportunities for learning and change. Finally, we examine specific principles that connect individual improvement projects to larger-scale organizational change, and we thus set the stage for case studies of health system improvement that are explored in subsequent chapters.

Change Concepts

The ability to design and to rapidly test change is an essential capacity of professional learning environments.[3,4] New design ideas—or certainly those with sufficient merit to be tested—arise from individual or collective reflection on processes now in place, with attention to high-leverage steps whose modification will enhance work quality and efficiency. In Chapter 2 we generated multiple ideas for change from perspectives inside the system. These perspectives (for example, of clinicians, nurses, receptionists, administrators, other stakeholders) provide necessary insight into the process of care as experienced by workers themselves in their very act of working. But these same participants can also step back and view their work from outside the processes. Imagine an industrial assembly line or workshop, and now imagine a catwalk or viewing deck that traverses this same space. Imagine, finally, the value to participants of moving back and forth, every day, between these parallel spaces, between the workstation where processes are known experientially and the viewing deck where those same processes are understood analytically. The opportunities for learning, making, and leading improvement are greatly enhanced by such perceptual shifts.[5]

DeBono has characterized this shifting of perspectives in greater detail, and has discovered in this reframing a rich source of underlying concepts that become generators of specific improvement ideas.[6] If we understand the underlying concept on which a specific idea is based, we can use this concept to brainstorm multiple new options for action. Health professionals will recognize in this formulation a restatement of clinical reasoning processes that become increasingly natural with growing experience. Consider the example in Sidebar 6-1 (page 83) that links underlying generic concepts to specific intervention ideas.

As the sidebar story and diagram both illustrate, when we travel a road or pursue an idea, we are likely to encounter junctions of choice for new and different paths. Once we have committed ourselves to a single idea, we risk narrowing our perspective to this one channel (as would have occurred, in our example, if Dr. Hart had insisted only on increasingly aggressive pharmacologic solutions). Although such single-minded commitment is sometimes quite appropriate, there is often more benefit to be derived from what DeBono calls "lateral thinking"—a form of reasoning that invites us to pull back to the underlying concept, to clarify this concept by naming it, and to then imagine alternate paths forward.[6]

Langley and colleagues have incorporated DeBono's underlying concepts into a framework that specifically supports improvement-oriented change. They have characterized these common pathways as *change concepts*, which they define as general categories or approaches to change that stimulate more specific improvement ideas.[7] A useful taxonomy of such change concepts has been developed, and Langley et al., have now identified 70 generic change concepts that can be applied to improvement design across a wide spectrum of work settings, including health care.

Indeed, change-concept thinking is well suited to the delivery and improvement of patient care. Experienced clinicians routinely apply taxonomies of diagnosis and inter-

vention, and reflective practitioners grow increasingly facile in movements left or right (backward and forward) along these clinical branches. The case in Sidebar 6-1 of cardiovascular risk reduction offers a most elementary example. At more sophisticated levels, such thinking can and should be built into formal process-focused quality improvement initiatives. (*See*, for example, the hip replacement case study described in the subsequent section.)

We offer ten core concepts here that have proven especially valuable in our own improvement work. (These concepts are further characterized in the case study and figures that follow, and specific examples also are provided in Table 6-1, page 86 and Table 6-2, page 88.) Readers might find that these terms give a name to changes that have already been locally identified, or they might help to clarify thinking about where in the local process new changes should be initiated. Remember, however, that change concepts cannot serve as a substitute for serious thinking about local processes of care. If practitioners have information and clear ideas about where process improvement is required, this knowledge and judgment should be trusted. Change concepts can jump-start stalled thinking or redirect it, but of course they must never supplant that thinking. We invite readers to consider local application of the generic concepts shown in Figure 6-1 (page 84).

Case Example: Using Change Concepts to Improve Clinical Care for Hip Replacement

To illustrate the utility of change-concept thinking in quality innovation and cost reduction, we review the experience of a small group of orthopedic surgeons, nurses, and administrative support staff, who came together to improve clinical care of patients undergoing hip replacement. In the current case, core process analysis was guided by the Clinical Improvement Worksheet[8–10] and Clinical Value Compass Worksheet (*see* Chapters 3 and 4), and idea generation was enriched through explicit attention to underlying change concepts. We again remind readers (as in previous chapters) that improvement work is the responsibility of all health care workers and that it can be effectively implemented by either individual practitioners, informal professional groups (who work separately but in parallel), or well-coordinated multidisciplinary teams. The hip replacement clinicians chose a team-based approach, but in other settings both individuals and informal groups have found the use of change concepts to be similarly fruitful.

SIDEBAR 6-1. **Reducing Cardiovascular Risk**

Dr. Hart is re-evaluating Andrew Jones, a 45-year-old office manager with untreated hypertension and elevated serum cholesterol. Mr. Jones is 30 pounds overweight and acknowledges that both his stressful job and his troubled marriage distract him from self-care. He eats "on the run," sometimes skipping meals and then overcompensating with whatever junk food is available at the work cafeteria. At today's office visit, as during his prior visit, Mr. Jones's blood pressure is elevated to 155/90.

Dr. Hart is concerned about this blood pressure reading and about Mr. Jones's cardiovascular risk in general. She persuades Mr. Jones that his blood pressure needs to be reduced, and she invites him to brainstorm ideas that will support this goal. The "main route" along which they begin their brainstorming (route X in the figure below) is "blood pressure control" (or, even further upstream, general "cardiovascular risk reduction"). Together, they come up with several initial ideas:

A. Initiate an antihypertensive medication.
B. Begin an exercise routine at the local health club.
C. Join a work-based dietary counseling program.

Mr. Jones quickly selects option A, the antihypertensive medication, because he believes that this route will be simplest and most effective, with the least impact on his hectic schedule. However, at his follow-up appointment two months later, his blood pressure remains high despite compliance with the prescribed regimen, and he is experiencing unpleasant side effects from the medication. At this point, instead of pushing further down pathway A (another medication), Dr. Hart prudently "pulls back" to the underlying concept X, and suggests an alternate path forward: B (exercise regimen), C (dietary program), or even D (a new idea such as marital therapy or personal counseling to manage psychosocial stressors).

DeBono illustrates the value of a generic concept (X) and its relation to specific ideas (A, B, and C) as shown in the figure below. This model can be conceptualized as a path forward on main route, X, with three specific branch routes labeled "A," "B," and "C." Similarly, a core concept labeled "X" might lead to many ideas labeled "A," "B," and "C."[1]

Reference

1. De Bono E.: *Serious Creativity: Using the Power of Lateral Thinking to Create New Ideas*, 1st ed. New York City: Harper Business, 1992.

Change Concept–Idea Relationship

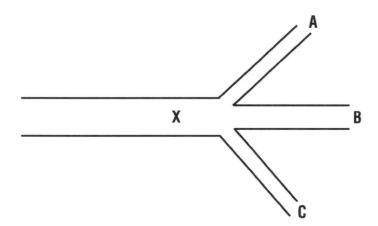

The change concept–idea relationship can be thought of as a core concept, X, which might lead to many ideas or branches, including A, B, and C.

FIGURE 6-1. **A Worksheet for Generating Specific Change Ideas**

If your thinking needs a jolt, select one or two of these change concepts to help identify an area or process for change and then design a specfic change.

Underlying generic change concepts   **My specific ideas are:**

1. Modify input.   _____

2. Combine steps.   _____

3. Eliminate failures at handoffs   _____
    between steps.

4. Eliminate a step.   _____

5. Reorder the sequence of steps.   _____

6. Change an element in the process   _____
    by creating an arrangement with   _____
    another party to change the   _____
    concept of the process.   _____

7. Replace a step with a better   _____
    value alternative.   _____

8. From knowledge of service or   _____
    product that is produced, redesign   _____
    production.   _____

9. From knowledge of use of service   _____
    or product, redesign product.   _____

10. With knowledge of need and aim,   _____
    redesign.   _____

Figure 6-1. Specific change ideas can be generated for generic change concepts.

---

① Outcomes → Select a Population

Using the Clinical Improvement Worksheet, the hip replacement team specified its aims with respect to achievement of clinical, functional, satisfaction, and cost outcomes that were superior to current outcomes.

② Process → Analyze the Process

By constructing a flow diagram, the hip replacement team analyzed caregiving processes that produced current results. This enabled the team to visualize specific steps in the provision of joint replacement care. Figure 6-2 (page 85) illustrates its high-level flowchart. Until this exercise was performed, no individual participant had been fully cognizant of the entire process of care. By stepping onto the "catwalk,"

however, and viewing their own work from the outside, team members now felt empowered to generate both general and specific ideas for improvement of care.

③ Changes → Generate Change Ideas

What ideas do we have for changing what's done (process) to get better results? As the hip replacement team constructed its high-level flowchart, several ideas emerged spontaneously for improvement of specific processes. The observation was made, for example, that certain clinicians initiated aggressive physical therapy very early in the presurgical process (to prepare the patient for surgery), whereas others waited until after the procedure to initiate this physical therapy. Might there be

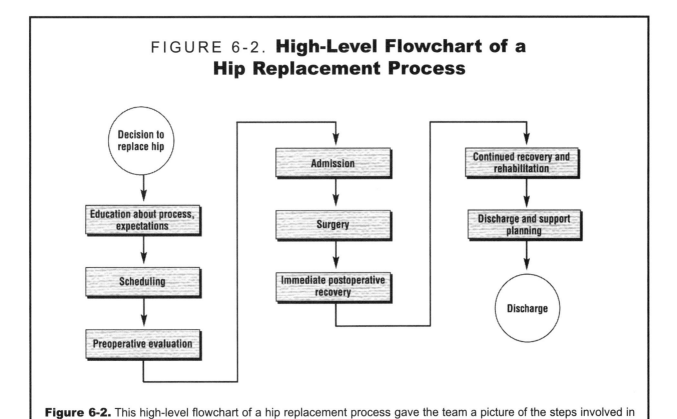

FIGURE 6-2. **High-Level Flowchart of a Hip Replacement Process**

Figure 6-2. This high-level flowchart of a hip replacement process gave the team a picture of the steps involved in providing joint replacement care.

value (increased quality, greater efficiency) in standardizing the timing of physical therapy referrals? These early ideas were recorded on a "potential changes" list. But after completing development of the high-level flowchart, and after marveling at the complexity of actual care process that this flowchart revealed, the team wished to broaden and to deepen its thinking about specific interventions before committing to a first PDSA cycle of change.

To optimize both efficiency and effectiveness of this critical third step on the Clinical Improvement Worksheet—"What ideas do we have for changing what's done (process) to get better results?"—the team worked through the following activities:

- All team members silently wrote down their improvement ideas, and they pinpointed each idea on the flowchart. These improvement ideas came from many sources: personal experience, professional knowledge, direct observation, literature review, and clinical benchmarking. (*See* Chapter 5.)
- Each participant created a simple two-column matrix, listing specific improvement ideas in the right-hand column and aligning these with underlying, generic change concepts listed in the left-hand

column. Table 6-1 (page 86) is an example of one team member's list.
- Pairs of team members discussed their specific ideas and corresponding generic change concepts, promoting greater clarity of the clinical process and a still larger list of improvement ideas. This was accomplished through use of the generic change concepts to stimulate lateral thinking, with specific application of the concepts either upstream or downstream from the original flowchart location.
- The team now generated a long master list of ideas, placing these all in an "idea pool" that generated much excitement among participants. Reflecting on this idea pool, team members came to believe that the current process of care was no longer an option, and they now had several very concrete ideas to test in the days ahead.

(Notice that the hip replacement team began with a *specific* idea, then stepped back to identify underlying change concepts, and finally used their insight from this dual perspective to generate many more specific ideas. Another valid approach is to begin with generic change concepts themselves, and to use these directly to initiate the brainstorming.)

TABLE 6-1. **Underlying Change Concepts for Specific Change Ideas**

Underlying, Generic Change Concepts	My Specific Ideas
Modify input	Start a physical conditioning program in advance of surgery to make our patients fit for the surgical procedure and thereby reduce risk and speed up recovery.
Combine steps	Bring together the preoperative workup and the basic laboratory work and make one step out of two.
Replace a step with a better value alternative	Save money by standardizing our decision making about which prosthesis to use and always selecting the lowest-cost, clinically appropriate prosthesis.

- Two participants then volunteered to take the ten top-ranked ideas for change—those voted most powerful or feasible by team members who had direct day-to-day knowledge of the working process—and to display them on a new high-level flowchart of their joint replacement care process. This enabled the entire team to visualize sites of greatest potential leverage, where specific pilot tests of change might yield greatest impact on outcomes and costs.

Figure 6-3 (page 87) illustrates the product of this last exercise and offers an especially practical formulation for design of change in clinical processes. All ten of our previously listed generic change concepts are identified and correlated with specific sites of potential change in the hip replacement process of care. In Table 6-2 (page 88), the ten points of intervention are described textually in greater detail. These same generic change concepts have been used repeatedly by individual practitioners and by formal improvement teams to stimulate efficient redesign and improvement in multiple patient care settings.

When the hip replacement team reviewed its work, several important but unanticipated benefits had been achieved, including the following:

- A "savings account" of great ideas had been built up, permitting individual team members (or smaller pairings of individuals, or the entire team) to pursue successive small tests of change over time—PDSA cycle 1, PDSA cycle 2, and so on.
- Deeper appreciation of the current process had been linked with very specific ideas for both improvement

of discrete elements within that process—incremental first-order change—and redesign of the entire process—innovation or second-order change.

- Ten powerful clinical change concepts had been explored in detail and could now be applied more regularly and thoroughly, not only in joint replacement care, but also in the management of other important orthopedic conditions.

Empowered by these general insights and specific ideas, the team quickly proceeded to Step 4 on the Clinical Improvement Worksheet: selecting a first test of change.

④ Pilot → Select a Change for Pilot Testing

How can we pilot test an improvement idea using the PDSA method? To select its first pilot test, participants reviewed the ten change ideas listed in Table 6-2 (page 88) and then asked, "Where is the leverage for change? What changes will have the largest effect on patient safety? On current resource use? On current reliability? On other subprocesses (including influence or ripple effects on the entire collection of interlinked subprocesses)?" Next, team members considered the relative complexity of pilot alternatives (illustrated in a "ramp of complexity" that has been described by Langley et al.[11]), and they addressed the critical question: "What is the largest feasible change that we can test, that we predict will lead to improvement, and that we can implement by a near, certain date?"

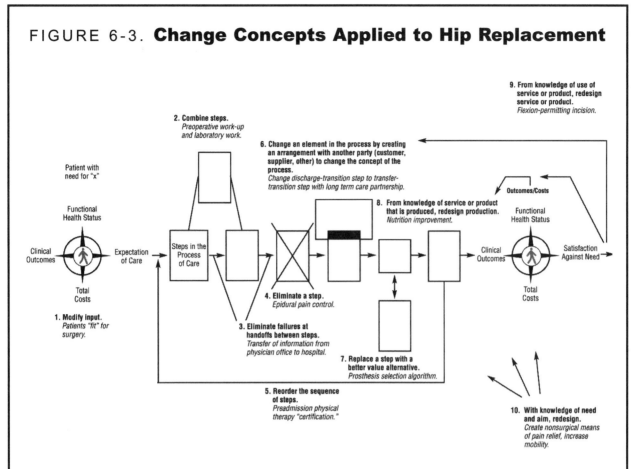

FIGURE 6-3. **Change Concepts Applied to Hip Replacement**

Figure 6-3. This figure shows how ten concepts for changing any process are applied to a hip replacement case. Generic change concepts, specific improvement ideas for changing the inputs, action steps, outcomes, and the entire process are superimposed on the core clinical process represented as a flowchart of hip replacement care. Examples of improvements in the value of hip joint replacement are shown in italics.

In light of these several considerations, the team elected to combine three ideas into a pilot test:

1. Procedure for getting the patient fit for surgery
2. Prosthesis-selection algorithm
3. Nutrition improvement

The remaining seven improvement ideas were held in the team's aforementioned "savings account" of high leverage ideas to be used in subsequent cycles of change.

Change in Organizations

For purposes of simple exposition, the hip replacement case study is presented as if in a vacuum, with only minimal discussion of the greater health care organization in which the improvement team functioned. But real-world improvement work does not occur in a vacuum. Health care organizations are complex systems, and practitioners of improvement must understand how change occurs within this context of greater complexity. How do local changes affect the larger organizational system, and how does that system "push back?" Such understanding is essential not only for implementation of change but also for its maintenance over time and for its successful adaptation in new settings. We conclude this chapter with a brief discussion of change within larger organizational contexts and offer two further exercises that support navigation through such workplace domains.

A Model for Change

Gustafson and colleagues have described a model of change implementation in organizational settings.[12] This model recognizes two sets of key actors: innovators and opinion leaders. The first group stimulates generation of (and experimentation with) new ideas, whereas the second group promotes diffusion of these ideas within the organization. There is no requirement for these functions to be

TABLE 6-2. **Change Concepts for Improving Hip Replacements**

Change Concept	Idea for Change
1. Modify input	Increase the patient's ability to successfully withstand the intervention and recover more quickly by operating on patients who have been brought to a higher level of personal fitness and better nutritional status before surgery.
2. Combine steps	Decrease the work and waste associated with doing things as multiple steps by combining the steps into a single step, such as combining the preoperative laboratory work and preoperative evaluation.
3. Eliminate failures at handoffs between steps	Couple steps with fewer errors by making the egress from one step become the explicit ingress to the next. For example, redesign the format of the discharge-planning forms and the orders for admission to home health and follow-up physical therapy care.
4. Eliminate a step	Stop doing things that do not add significant value to the desired result. For example, eliminate the need for epidural pain control by extending the use of the other analgesics.
5. Reorder steps	Achieve a smoother overall flow of care by placing a late step in an earlier position in the process. For example, have the physical therapist teach patients to manage their own postoperative rehabilitation care before admission when they are alert, in no postoperative pain, and ready to learn.
6. Change an element in the process by creating an arrangement with another party	Create a new process altogether by combining a step with something extrinsic to the current process. For example, combine discharge with admission to a transition care setting, thus making the discharge step into a transfer step.
7. Replace a step with a better value alternative	Identify a better method or technology to perform a given step, such as using a decision algorithm for prosthesis selection that results in a recommendation for the lowest-cost, clinically appropriate device.
8. From knowledge of service or product produced, redesign production	Redesign the process when the full nature of the result and its possible contributors are known, such as creating optimal nutritional status before surgery after recognizing the value of good nutritional status for prompt healing.
9. From knowledge of use of service or product, redesign service or product	Facilitate consideration of further process changes by knowing the next use of the end result of the process. For example, create a flexion-permitting incision for the joint replacement after recognizing the need for early ambulation.
10. With knowledge of need and aim, redesign	Consider and design entirely different services if the need is clearly known. For example, develop alternative approaches to achieving pain relief, with or without the intervening surgery, when the need for pain relief is clarified as the purpose of the intervention.

served by the same individual, and indeed they typically are not. Innovators might be relatively new to the organization (though of course this is not always the case), and it is often this fresh and even "foreign" perspective that permits creativity to flourish. Opinion leaders are more likely to have served for a longer time within the same organization, and to have gained colleagues' respect and attention by virtue of this longevity (again a generalization). Healthy organizations benefit from the creative tension of these complementary (and co-occurring) functions of innovation, modeling, and diffusion.

Gustafson et al., suggest that these actors (and other players in the organization) are driven toward improvement in a context of tension for change—the belief that the organization must change in order to survive or to prosper. As depicted in Figure 6-4 (below), the key actors must perceive that a superior alternative (an improvement) exists and that the social support and technical competence (skills and self-efficacy) are available to manage the change process and to achieve desired results. With these essential elements in place, the organization can commit itself to change and can plan for it. The improvement cycle is thus entered; change can be implemented

and monitored, with results fed back to participants to support further commitment and planning.

Creating Change

Whereas Gustafson's insights arise from the examination of successful organizational change, John P. Kotter has studied changes that failed. By exploring the underlying causes of such failure, Kotter identifies essential leadership qualities that support an organization's achievement of meaningful change. His important work, *Leading Change,*[13] describes eight stages in the process of improvement leadership. The reader will recognize in Kotter's eight-stage model several similarities to the clinical improvement strategy we have promoted in earlier chapters of the present text. His model includes the following phases:

1. Establish a sense of urgency.
2. Create a guiding coalition.
3. Develop a vision and strategy.
4. Communicate the change vision.
5. Empower broad-based action.
6. Generate short-term wins.
7. Consolidate gains, and produce more change.
8. Anchor new approaches in the culture.

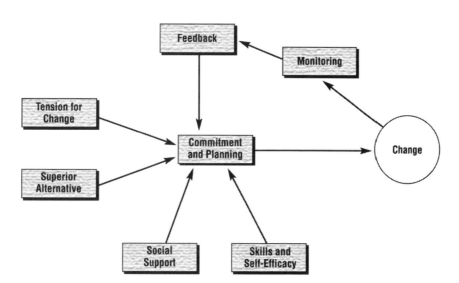

FIGURE 6-4. **A Model of Organizational and Individual Change**

Figure 6-4. This diagram illustrates how successful change occurs when a combination of political, social, administrative, and rational processes are put in place. Used with permission from *Systems to Support Health Policy Analysis: Theory, Models, and Uses* by David Gustafson, et al. Chicago: Health Administration Press, 1992, p. 45.

The tools we have presented in earlier chapters of this text can support practitioners' improvement work in each of Kotter's eight stages.

Practitioners can prepare themselves for introduction of improvement ideas into clinical organizations. On the basis of specific challenges identified during current or past improvement projects, think through Kotter's eight-stage model and identify actions that might facilitate the leading of organizational change.

Steps	Possible Actions
1. Establish a sense of urgency by	
□ identifying the "best anywhere" and the gap between yours and theirs	
□ identifying the consequences of being less than the best	
□ exploring sources of complacency	
2. Create a guiding coalition to	
□ find the right people	
□ create trust	
□ share common goal	
3. Develop a vision and strategy that is	
□ easily pictured	
□ attractive	
□ feasible	
□ clear	
□ flexible	
□ communicable	
4. Communicate the change vision in a way that	
□ is simple	
□ uses metaphor	
□ works in multiple forums	
□ involves doing instead of telling	
□ explains inconsistencies	
□ involves give and take	
5. Empower broad-based action by	
□ communicating sensible vision to employees	
□ making organization's structures compatible with action	
□ providing needed training	
□ aligning information and human resource systems	
□ confronting supervisors who undercut change	
6. Generate short-term wins by	
□ fixing the date of certain change	
□ doing the easy stuff first	
□ using measurement to confirm change	
7. Consolidate gains and produce more change by	
□ identifying true interdependencies and smooth interconnections	
□ eliminating unnecessary dependencies	
□ identifying linked subsequent cycles of change	
8. Anchor new approaches in the culture with	
□ results	
□ conversation	
□ turnover	
□ succession	

Resistance to Change: A Marker of Identity?

Although the Gustafson et al. and Kotter models accurately characterize essential players and processes in organizational change, most of us can recount experiences when even obvious tension for change was insufficient to motivate key players within a system. What is the source of this internal resistance?

We suggest that both individuals and organizations are keenly sensitive to challenges to their own identity, and that perceived perturbations to the integrity of this identity—the introduction of material that is "strange" or "foreign"—might naturally trigger a self-protective response. This identity-preserving action is common to all living organisms and systems and is well illustrated in the familiar antigen-antibody response. When presented with an antigenic challenge, our bodies typically recognize the offending agent as foreign, and our immune cells generate specific antibodies to neutralize the threat. Although the defensive function of this antibody response is apparent to all who study cellular systems, we emphasize here that the same response also serves as a biologic expression of *self-identity*. In the very act of preserving its own boundary between self and other, the organism defines this boundary more precisely.

In similar fashion, when individuals and organizations express resistance to change, they could well be communicating a need to preserve the integrity of boundaries against potentially threatening, and certainly "foreign," ideas or interventions. The resistance itself might initially frustrate champions of change and innovation, but as in the case of molecular antibodies, this defense also sends a potentially valuable signal of self-identity. Skilled leaders of change, when sensitive to such signals, can use them to better explore the system itself, and this exploration might in turn support change strategies that can be embraced by all participants. The message for practitioners of clinical improvement is therefore that resistance, when encountered, should not be resisted in turn. Rather, it should be examined, understood, and actively engaged.

Practical Barriers to Change

The probing of a system's resistance, as just suggested, might reveal previously unacknowledged priorities, fears, and expectations. It will also likely expose very practical challenges, including perceived insufficiency of resources and inadequacy of data. As suggested in Table 6-3 (below), however, even these seemingly straightforward barriers might be based upon assumptions that have not been fully articulated. Such barriers can be anticipated, and the

TABLE 6-3. Manifestations of Barriers to Change

Real-Life Barriers to Change	Manifested As
Inertia of current work	• Good people are really pretty busy. • There are too many committees already. • It's hard to even find a time to meet.
Managing the process of change	• Where do you start? • How can we hold the gains? • People are always coming and going • What data will be helpful, and how shall we get them? • What shall we do about those who aren't interested in changing?
Knowledge we don't have	• What does the patient think about this? • How do we proceed when the science is uncertain? • In the absence of our own data reflecting our own management of all our patients, how should we offer real information about risks and choices to our patients?
Things we underestimate and wish were easier to change	• Computer systems. • Getting administrative support. • Changing administrative work.

TABLE 6-4. **Reflective Questions to Facilitate Management of Barriers to a Change Idea**

Change Idea: _____

1. Do we have adequate tension for change?

   Sources of Tension from:
   □ Current waste
   □ Current external threats
   □ Known (and named) gaps in cost, service, and satisfaction
   □ Clear risks from continuing current practices

How might inadequate tension for change show up as resistance to our proposed change?

_____

_____

2. Is our alternative actionable? Does it seem sensible and possible?
   □ Is the alternative recognizable? Can people see themselves in the new work?
   □ Is the alternative explicitly aligned with the organization's culture?
   □ Has a sufficient change reserve been established?

If our coworkers don't see our proposed change as being able to implement, how might that manifest itself as resistance to change?

_____

_____

3. Do we have the improvement knowledge and skills needed to design and conduct the change?

   Improvement Knowledge:
   □ Do we have measures to learn and confirm that changes equal improvement?
   □ Do we have the ability to design and test rapid cycles and pilots of change?
   □ Do we have process and system pictures of work?
   □ Do we know our patients, customers, and beneficiaries?
   □ Do we understand variation within processes?

If we don't have the improvement knowledge that we need, how might that show up as resistance to our proposed changes?

_____

_____

   People Knowledge:
   □ Do we have the people knowledge to design and conduct change?
   □ Do we understand the sources of pride in work?
   □ Do we each have a personal vision for the future?

If we don't have the people knowledge that we need, how might that manifest itself as resistance to change?

_____

_____

Knowledge of Change Management:
☐ Do we know what we need to know about managing change?
☐ Do we have a clear aim and plan with known coalitions?
☐ Are resources assessed and is the agenda formulated?
☐ Do we have cycles of review, refinement, and consolidation of aim?
☐ Do we know what is not to change?
☐ Do we have a date certain for action?

If we don't have the knowledge of change management that we need, how might that show up as resistance to change?

_____

_____

Professional Knowledge:
☐ Do we have the professional and technical knowledge to design and conduct this change?
☐ Do we have subject knowledge?
☐ Do we have knowledge of the discipline?
☐ Do we have knowledge of the values relevant to this change?

If we don't have the professional and technical knowledge we need, how will it show up as resistance to change?

_____

_____

4. Do we have the social support necessary to undertake this change?
☐ Has an able and willing sponsor been identified?
☐ Have we anticipated resistance?
☐ What traditions, habits, activities, and policies support change?

If we don't have adequate social support, how will that show up as resistance to change?

_____

_____

5. Given all of the above, what are the implications for our actions?

_____

_____

6. Have any of these issues surfaced before?

_____

assumptions more deeply explored. When considering specific change ideas, the reflective questions listed in Table 6-4 (*see* pages 92–93) might facilitate practices' effective management of practical barriers.

Building on Change

In a world that itself is continually changing, the survival of health care systems depends on their capacity to stimulate and manage internal change. Clinicians not only must anticipate but indeed should embrace and strive to lead such inevitable transitions, whether these occur in direct patient care, in professional development, or in continuous improvement of health care delivery systems.

The current chapter has explored higher-order manifestations of change as these appear in health care settings. It has introduced both generic change concepts (that underlie specific improvement ideas) and models of change promotion (and resistance) in larger organizations. In Chapters 7 and 9, we explore the maintenance of such change in increasingly complex systems of care. How do we sustain our gains, and how do we extend them? In Chapter 8 we link these clinical and system changes to the developmental transitions of practitioners themselves. What processes and structures support clinicians' growing competence as agents and leaders of change? These are not simple questions, and we can't provide simple, one-size-fits-all answers. But the well-being of our patients, and the need to improve the quality and safety of our health care delivery systems, require earnest exploration and intelligent action.

References

1. Personal communication between the author [P.B.B.] and John Kelsch, Chief Quality Officer, Xerox Corporation, Stamford, CT, 1992.
2. Schön D.A.: *The Reflective Practitioner: How Professionals Think in Action.* New York City: Basic Books, 1983.
3. Argyris C., Schön D.A.: *On Organizational Learning II.* Reading, MA: Addison-Wesley, 1996.
4. Kolb D.A., Rubin I.M.: *Organizational Behavior: An Experiential Approach.* Englewood Cliffs, NJ: Prentice-Hall, 1991.
5. Parks S.D: *Leadership Can Be Taught: A Bold Approach for a Complex World.* Boston: Harvard Business School Press, 2005.
6. De Bono E.: *Serious Creativity: Using the Power of Lateral Thinking to Create New Ideas.* New York City: Harper Business, 1992.
7. Langley G.J., et al.: *The Improvement Guide: A Practical Approach to Enhancing Organizational Performance.* San Francisco: Jossey-Bass Publishers, 1996
8. Nelson E., et al.: Improving Health Care, Part 2: A Clinical Improvement Worksheet and Users' Manual. *Jt Comm J Qual Improv* 22:531–548, Aug. 1996.
9. Nelson E., et al.: Improving Health Care, Part 3: Clinical benchmarking for best patient care. *Jt Comm J Qual Improv* 22:599–616, Sep. 1996.
10. Nelson E., et al.: Improving Health Care, Part 1: The Clinical Value Compass. *Jt Comm J Qual Improv* 22:243–258, Apr. 1996.
11. Langley G.J., Nolan K.M., Nolan T.W.: The foundation of improvement. *Quality Progress* 27:81–86, Jun. 1994.
12. Gustafson D.H., Cats-Baril W.L., Alemi F.: *Systems to Support Health Policy Analysis: Theory, Models, and Uses.* Ann Arbor, MI: Health Administration Press, 1992.
13. Kotter J.P.: *Leading Change.* Boston: Harvard Business School Press, 1996.

SUSTAINING AND EXTENDING CLINICAL IMPROVEMENTS: A HEALTH SYSTEM'S USE OF CLINICAL PROGRAMS TO BUILD QUALITY INFRASTRUCTURE

Brent C. James, Joel S. Lazar

The aim of this book is transformation of the style of American management. Transformation of American style of management is not a job of reconstruction, nor is it revision. It requires a whole new structure, from the foundation upward. —W.E. Deming[1(p. ix)]

Successful optimization of health care delivery requires not only that we strive continually to improve the processes and outcomes of our daily work but also that we build in strategies to sustain those improvements once achieved and that we extend successes to other work settings inside and outside our own organization. Many practitioners of improvement have seen their initial successes fail to take hold in the long term, or fail to spread to other colleagues and practice sites. Such failure of sustainability has immediate consequences for patient care. Less obviously, but also importantly, enthusiasm for future quality improvement initiatives might diminish as well.

Inspired by Deming's transformation of American management, many health care leaders are trying to transform American medicine as well. Here, too, a whole new structure is required, "from the foundation upward." If our goal is to successfully promote quality in health care systems and to sustain it, new models of both frontline care and organizational infrastructure must be designed, tested, and refined. This chapter offers an extended case study of one health care system that has created and implemented such a model.

The quality management pioneer, Joseph Juran, identified three core elements of a comprehensive quality-based strategy (the "Quality Trilogy"):[2]

1. Quality design (or quality planning) identifies the needs of individuals who are served by the organization and establishes strategies to meet those needs through development of better products and services.

2. Quality improvement generates methods to continually reassess prioritized targets and innovatively refine product and service delivery.

3. Quality control builds improved services into usual operations, via core data flow and management infrastructure, to sustain ongoing processes.

Previous chapters in the present book have focused especially on the first two components of Juran's Quality Trilogy. Indeed, the generation of change ideas and concepts (Chapters 2 and 6), the use of Clinical Improvement Worksheets and Clinical Value Compasses (Chapters 3 and 4), and the process of benchmarking (Chapter 5) are all practices of quality design and improvement. We have suggested, as well, that improvement works best when it is built into daily work flow processes. This latter feature does indeed contribute to Juran's third component, quality control, but in isolation it does not ensure that such control will be sustained in the long term.

The current chapter reviews the experience of one regional health system, Intermountain Healthcare, as it has endeavored during the past decade to sustain early improvements and to build a sophisticated quality management program that integrates design, improvement, and control of best-care processes. Readers will note that the present discussion shifts our perspective from previous chapters' presentations, but attention remains focused on a common theme. Whereas we previously introduced basic concepts and exercises, which we then illustrated with specific case examples, here we let the case discussion itself take center stage, and we augment this narrative with sidebar references to core quality principles addressed earlier in the volume. Our purpose is to demonstrate what the whole system looks like when basic improvement ideas are integrated seamlessly in advanced applications.

We shall see that although quality improvement (QI) and innovation are often generated at the frontline microsystems of care, quality design and control (that is, the planning, maintenance, and extension of improvements over time) often depend on committed mesosystem support as well. Intermountain's data communication systems and quality management infrastructure have promoted improvements in both system performance and patient outcomes. In addition, the integration of quality design, improvement, and control has enabled this organization to generate reliable new clinical knowledge from frontline care delivery experiences and to rapidly deploy new research findings across care delivery locations.

A Case Study: The Intermountain Healthcare System and the Clinical Program Approach

Intermountain Healthcare is an integrated, nonprofit health system serving the needs of Utah and southeastern Idaho residents. The system includes 21 hospitals, 100-plus outpatient clinics, and 26,000 employees (including 1,250 core physicians and approximately 2,000 associated physi-

cians)[3] Intermountain was an early innovator and adapter of formal QI methods, and the system documented several early successes.[4,5] Although these experiences confirmed that Deming's process management methods could be applied to health care delivery, they also highlighted a major challenge: Initial results were difficult to sustain and even more difficult to extend beyond local settings. Success in one location did not lead to widespread adoption, even among Intermountain's own facilities.

Since the quality movement's inception, most care delivery organizations have focused exclusively on improvement. Few systems, however, have built a comprehensive quality framework that integrates this improvement work with preplanning design and postdevelopment control. In 1996, Intermountain began to implement such an integrated program across its many inpatient and outpatient practices. The program depends on effective communication between frontline (microsystem) units of care—where new change ideas are generated and implemented on the basis of needs and experiences of patients and clinical staff—and systemwide quality management infrastructure (mesosystem)—where larger-scale resources support and coordinate frontline efforts. (*See* Sidebar 7-1, below, for further discussion of microsystems and mesosystems of care.)

At the microsystem level, Intermountain's therapeutic strategies depend heavily on a new "shared baselines"

SIDEBAR 7-1. Core Quality Principle: Microsystems and Mesosystems of Care

As discussed in Chapter 1, microsystems are the small, naturally occurring frontline units that provide most clinical care to most people. These units are characterized in terms of functional processes, patterns of communication, and the skill sets of each participant.[1] "Collections" of frontline clinical microsystems form mesosytems of care that might serve patients with specific needs, integrating sequential processes and supporting parallel clinical units across the care continuum.

Intermountain Health's Clinical Programs, described in the current chapter, combine microsystem principles and practices with Deming's original idea to "organize everything around value-added high-priority work

processes."[2] This organization permits geographic extension of value-based microsystem structures, yielding new forms of mesosystem support that are greater than the sum of their parts. By focusing on the high-priority activities common to local sites, Intermountain's Clinical Programs build value-based infrastructure across frontline microsystems with similar caregiving and outcome tracking needs.

References
1. Nelson E.C., et al.: Microsystems in health care: Part 1. Learning from high-performing front- line clinical units. *Jt Comm J Qual Improv* 28:472–493, Sep. 2002.
2. Personal communication with the author [B.C.J.] and W.E. Demming, Ph.D., independent consultant, Washington, DC, 1996.

approach to care delivery. This model evolved during early QI projects as a mechanism to functionally implement evidence-based medicine:[6] All health professionals associated with a particular clinical work process (for example, physicians, nurses, pharmacists, therapists, technicians, administrators) come together as a functional team. Participants build an evidence-based, best-practice guideline, fully understanding that it will not perfectly fit any one patient in the real care delivery setting. The team blends this guideline into clinical work flow, using standard order sets, clinical worksheets, and other similar tools. On implementation, health professionals adapt their shared common approach to the needs of each individual patient. Across more than 30 implemented clinical shared baselines, 5% to 15% of the content of a shared baseline is typically modified by Intermountain's physicians and nurses to meet the specific needs of a particular patient. The presence of such baselines makes it "easy to do things right,"[7] that is, according to clinical guidelines, while relying on practitioners' expertise to manage exceptional circumstances. This approach also contributes to efficiency, as skilled clinicians can focus their attention on a subset of critical issues, trusting that the remainder of the care process is reliable. These same shared baselines also facilitate structuring of the electronic data system, greatly enhancing the effectiveness of automated clinical information. Arguably, shared baselines are the key to successful implementation of electronic medical record systems. (*See* Sidebar 7-2, below, for discussion of shared baselines as a form of high-leverage change concept.)

At the mesosystem level, Intermountain has designed a clinical program model that clarifies and rationalizes a self-aware, self-sustaining quality infrastructure, connecting functionally related clinical units from across the care continuum. Construction of the mesosystem featured the following four major elements:

1. Key process analysis
2. An outcomes tracking system, which measures and reports accurate and timely medical, cost, and patient satisfaction results
3. An organizational structure to use outcomes data to hold practitioners accountable and to enable measured progress on shared clinical goals
4. Aligned incentives to harvest some portion of resulting cost savings back to the care delivery organization. (This last feature is often overlooked in quality systems but it is essential to achieve sustained buy-in from participants. Although in many instances better quality can demonstrably reduce total care delivery costs, current payment mechanisms direct most such savings to health care payers rather than to providers who have actually achieved the cost reductions.)

SIDEBAR 7-2. Core Quality Principle: Change Concepts

Intermountain Healthcare's "shared baseline" derives from Womack, Jones, and Roos' powerful concept of "mass customization,"[1] a process through which infrastructure for change is built directly into work operations. Performance variation is tracked and analyzed routinely within this system, and is fed back into a learning model that regularly supports new strategies for change. Although both the Womack, Jones, and Roos concept and Intermountain's clinical adaptation were developed before the Langley, et al.,[2] term change concept, the principle of shared baselines serves precisely this idea-stimulating role within Intermountain's organization.

As described in Chapter 6, change concepts are general categories or approaches to change that stimulate more specific improvement ideas. The utility of such concepts resides in their capacity to generate broadly applicable solutions that remain specific in their implementation. The high-leverage change concept of shared baselines or process standardization facilitates both work flow efficiency and quality monitoring, while justifying and structuring Intermountain's electronic medical record. A single idea thus promotes multiple ideas, with impacts on quality design, improvement, and control that are manifest throughout the clinical system.

References
1. Womack J., Jones D., Roos D.: *The Machine That Changed the World.* New York City: Harper Collins, 1991.
2. Langley G.J., et al.: *The Improvement Guide: A Practical Approach to Enhancing Organizational Performance.* San Francisco: Jossey-Bass, 1996.

In the remainder of this chapter, we address the first three of these clinical program elements, with special attention to care process models (CPMs), which link well-defined population-based mesosystem structures with clinical processes at the front line of care.

Key Process Analysis: Identifying and Analyzing the Fundamental Work of a Health System

The Institute of Medicine's prescription for reform of U.S. health care noted that an effective system should be organized around its most common elements.[8] Each year for four years, Intermountain attempted to identify high-priority clinical conditions for coordinated action through expert consensus among senior clinical and administrative leaders using formal Delphi methods. Despite a seemingly successful consensus process, however, leaders remained focused primarily on their own departmental priorities, and meaningfully coordinated action was not achieved. In 1996, Intermountain therefore moved from expert consensus to objective measurement, in which analytic methods would be used to identify and prioritize frontline work processes.

To facilitate this complex task, Intermountain's strategic clinical planners subdivided Intermountain's operations into four large classes:

1. Work processes centered around specific clinical conditions

2. Clinical work processes that are not condition-specific but that support clinical services (for example, processes located within pharmacy, pathology, anesthesiology/ procedure rooms, nursing units, intensive care units, patient safety)

3. Processes associated with patient satisfaction

4. Administrative support processes (for example, billing, human resources, informatics)

Within each category, the analytic team attempted to identify all major work processes that produced value-added results. (*See also* Sidebar 7-3, below, for discussion of process analysis.)

Intermountain planners then prioritized the work processes. To illustrate, within clinical conditions, the planning team performed the following actions:

1. Measured the number of patients affected

2. Estimated clinical risk to the patient. Intensity of care served as a surrogate for clinical risk, with care intensity measured as cost per case. This produced results that had high face validity with both frontline clinicians and administrative leadership.

3. Measured base-state variability within a particular clinical work process by calculating the coefficient of variation, based on intensity of care (cost per case)

4. Used Batalden and Nelson's concept of clinical microsystems (*see* Chapter 1 of this volume and Sidebar 7-1, page 96) to identify specialty groups that routinely worked together on the basis of shared patients and shared processes for managing those patients.[9,10] This was a key element for organizational structure.

5. Used expert judgment to identify underserved populations (the ethical principle of social justice) and to balance the roll-out across all elements of the Intermountain care delivery system

Among more than 1,000 initial inpatient and outpatient condition-based clinical work processes, only 104 of

---

SIDEBAR 7-3. Core Quality Principle: Process Analysis

As discussed in Chapter 2, the work of quality improvement—and also quality design and control—begins with thoughtful identification and clarification of all clinical and administrative processes that are pertinent to actual patient care. This reflective activity might be initiated via survey of participating "players" or via detailed mapping of local processes. When key elements have been identified, formal analytic assessment of service frequency, intensity, and cost is essential to estab-

lish a common agenda that all participants can follow. Intermountain Healthcare has used all these approaches, most especially analytic assessment, to better characterize its own fundamental work processes. The result is deep understanding (in both quantitative and qualitative terms) of clinical operations, facilitating effective resource utilization, quality planning, and project prioritization. (*See* text of current chapter for specific details.)

these processes accounted for almost 95% of all of Intermountain's care delivery. Instead of the traditional 80/20 rule (that is, the Pareto principle, which stipulates that about 80% of results arise from about 20% of all causes), Intermountain saw a 90/10 rule. Patient results and costs of operations were massively concentrated within a relatively small number of high-priority clinical processes. Intermountain then addressed these processes in priority order to achieve the most good for the most patients, while freeing resources to enable traditional, one-by-one care delivery plans for uncommon clinical conditions.

Outcomes Tracking: Developing a Data System to Support Care Delivery and to Monitor Outcomes

Intermountain had tried twice before to start a formal program for clinical management supported by data monitoring and feedback. The effort failed each time, with significant financial and staffing consequences. When asked to make a third attempt, the Intermountain planning team first performed a careful "autopsy" on the first two attempts. This investigation revealed that on each previous attempt, clinicians had indeed stepped forward to take the lead on clinical management. In each case, however, Intermountain's planners uncritically assumed that these new clinical leaders could simply use the same administrative, cost-based data to manage clinical processes as had traditionally been used to manage hospital departments and to generate insurance claims. On careful examination, the administrative data contained gaping holes relevant to clinical care delivery. Moreover, the data were organized for facilities management, not patient management. New sets of measures more appropriate to clinical care were required.

One of the first activities of the National Quality Forum (NQF) on its creation in 1999 was to convene an expert panel (a Strategic Framework Board; SFB) to develop formal, evidence-based methods for the identification of valid measurement sets in clinical care.[11] The SFB found that outcomes tracking systems work best when designed around, and integrated into, frontline care delivery. Although frontline–integrated data systems can "roll up" into accountability reports for clinicians, clinical practice groups, hospitals, regions, care delivery systems, states, and the nation, the opposite is not true: data systems designed "top down" for national reporting usually cannot generate "bottom up" information flow necessary for process management and improvement at the point of care.[12] Such top-down systems often compete for limited

frontline resources, damaging care delivery at the patient interface.[13]

Intermountain adopted the NQF's data system design method. This approach begins with an evidence-based, best-practice guideline, laid out for care delivery (the shared baseline model, as described). Such baselines permit identification and testing of a comprehensive set of medical, cost, and satisfaction outcome measures, and enable generation of corresponding reports designed for clinical process management and improvement. The reports lead to a list of data elements and coding manuals, which in turn generate "data marts" within an electronic data warehouse. The result is an integrated medical record system that can merge patient registries with decision support tools, facilitating both point-of-care intervention and aggregated outcomes tracking. (*See also* Sidebar 7-4, page 100, for discussion of outcome measurement.)

The production of new clinical outcomes tracking data represented a significant investment for Intermountain. Therefore, addressing clinical work processes in priority order, as determined by key process analysis (described above), was critical. Initial progress was swift. For example, in 1997 Intermountain completed outcomes tracking systems for their two biggest clinical processes. Pregnancy, labor, and delivery represented 11% of Intermountain's total clinical volume. Ischemic heart disease represented another 10%. At the end of the year, Intermountain had a detailed clinical "dashboard" in place for approximately 21% of the system's total care delivery. The data system was designed for frontline process management, which was then rolled up into region- and system-level accountability reports. Today, outcomes data cover almost 80% of Intermountain's inpatient and outpatient clinical care. Such data are immediately available through internal Web sites, with data lag times under one month in all cases, and a few days in most cases.

Organizational Structure: Building Relationships to Manage and to Improve Care Delivery Across the Care Continuum by Establishing Clinical Programs

When Intermountain started to develop new clinical programs, about two-thirds of their core physicians were community-based, independent practitioners. The structural reality of regional care necessitated a system of organization that heavily emphasized shared professional values, backed up by aligned financial incentives. (Notably, the program's early success relied exclusively on shared profes-

---

SIDEBAR 7-4. Core Quality Principle: Balanced Outcomes Measurement

We emphasize repeatedly in this volume the critical role of outcomes measurement in directing and refining quality performance. As primarily described in Chapter 4, the Clinical Value Compass maps patient outcomes in the important domains of clinical status, functional capacity, satisfaction against need, and (direct and indirect) costs.[1,2] Leaders at Intermountain Healthcare have used a similar classification scheme, combining the two value compass "directions" of clinical and functional status in a single "medical" domain. This becomes one corner of a conceptual triangle (rather than a four-directional compass), whose other two points are (as in the Clinical Value Compass) satisfaction and cost.[3-5] Of course, the precise labeling of different axes is less important than the broadly inclusive conception of outcomes that the Clinical Value Compass and Intermountain's own tracking system have in common. In both cases, identification and monitoring of a balanced set of outcomes enables clinicians to design, implement, and sustain meaningful improvements that all stakeholders can recognize as important.

References

1. Nelson E.C., et al.: Improving health care, Part 2: A Clinical Improvement Worksheet and users' manual. *Jt Comm J Qual Improv* 22:531–548, Aug. 1996.
2. Nelson E.C., et al.: Improving health care, Part 1: The Clinical Value Compass. *Jt Comm J Qual Improv* 22:243–258, Apr. 1996.
3. James B.C.: Information system concepts for quality measurement. *Med Care* 41:I71–I78, Jan. 2003.
4. James B.C.: Outcomes measurement. In: *Bridging the Gap Between Theory and Practice.* Chicago: Hospital Research and Education Trust (American Hospital Association), 1994, pp. 1–34.
5. James B.C.: Good enough? Standards and measurement in continuous quality improvement. In *Bridging the Gap Between Theory and Practice.* Chicago: Hospital Research and Education Trust (American Hospital Association), 1992, pp. 1–24.

---

sional values; financial incentives evolved quite late in the process and were always modest in size.)

The microsystem focus of the key process analysis (as described previously) provided the core organizational structure. Families of related processes, called clinical programs, identified care teams that routinely worked together, even though they often spanned traditional subspecialty boundaries (Figure 7-1, page 101). These related care teams represented the informal clinical mesosystem that took steps to organize and formalize. (*See* Sidebar 7-1, page 96, for discussion of microsystems and mesosystems of care.) Intermountain hired part-time physician leaders for each clinical program in each of its three major regions (Urban North, Urban Central, and Urban South), each region a network of outpatient practices and small community hospitals, organized around a large tertiary medical center. Physician leaders were required to practice actively within their clinical programs, to have the respect of their professional peers, and to complete formal training in clinical quality improvement methods through Intermountain's internal clinical improvement training program. (This "Advanced Training Program in Clinical Practice Improvement" is now open to external medical leaders, through Intermountain's collaboration with the Institute for Healthcare Improvement. Information is available at http://www.ihi.org/IHI/Programs/ConferencesAndTraining/AdvancedTrainingProgram.)

Recognizing that the bulk of clinical process management efforts rely on clinical staff, not just physicians, Intermountain also hired full-time "clinical operations administrators." Most of these clinical operations leaders (who support the clinical program leaders) are experienced nurse administrators. The resulting leadership dyad—a physician leader and a nursing/support staff leader—meets each month with every local team in its clinical program. They present and review patient outcomes and performance results, with attention to peer and national benchmark comparisons. (*See also* Chapter 5 on clinical benchmarking.) Attention is given to systemwide clinical improvement goals, tracking progress, identifying barriers, and discussing possible solutions. Within each region, all clinical program dyads meet monthly with their administrative counterparts (regional hospital administration, finance, information technology, insurance partners, nursing, and quality management). They review current clinical results, track progress on goals, and assign resources to overcome implementation barriers at the local level.

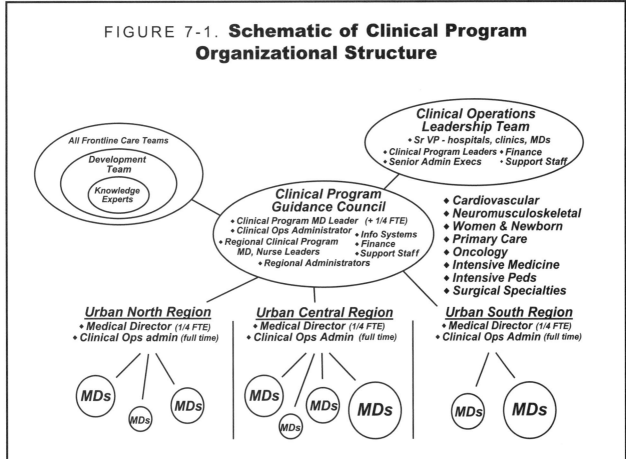

FIGURE 7-1. **Schematic of Clinical Program Organizational Structure**

Figure 7-1. Clinical Programs identified care teams, such as primary care practices, endocrinology practices, and inpatient medical unit, that routinely worked together. These related care teams represented the informal clinical mesosystem that took steps to organize and formalize.

In addition to their regional activities, all leaders within a particular clinical program (from across the entire Intermountain system) meet together monthly as a central guidance council. One of the three regional physician leaders is funded for an additional part-time role to oversee and coordinate the systemwide effort. Each system-level clinical program also has a separate, full-time clinical operations administrator. Finally, each guidance council is assigned at least one full-time statistician and at least one full-time data manager to help coordinate clinical outcomes data flow, produce outcomes tracking reports, and to perform special analyses. This structure coordinates a large part of Intermountain's existing staff support functions, such as medical informatics (electronic medical records), electronic data warehouse, finance, and purchasing, to assist the clinical management effort.

By design, each guidance council oversees a set of condition-based clinical work processes, as identified and

prioritized during the aforementioned key process analysis step. Each key clinical process is managed by a development team (Table 7-1, pages 100–101), which reports to the guidance council. Development teams meet each month. The majority of development team members are drawn from frontline physicians and clinical staff, geographically balanced across the Intermountain system, who have hands-on experience with the clinical care under discussion.[1] Development team members carry the team's activities—analysis and management system results—back to their frontline colleagues to seek their input and to help with implementation and operations. Each development team also has a designated physician leader, as well as "knowledge experts" drawn from each region. knowledge experts are usually specialists associated with the team's particular care process. For example, the Primary Care Clinical Program includes a Diabetes Mellitus Development Team (among others). Most team members are frontline primary care physicians and nurses

TABLE 7-1.

Intermountain Clinical Program and Development Teams*

Clinical Program
   Development Teams   Date started
      CPMs

Cardiovascular
   IHD Development Team   Jan. 1998
      AMI
   CHF Development Team   Jan. 2001
   CV Surgery Development Team   Jan. 1998
      Fast-track extubation
      Intra- and post-op glucose control
   Cardiac Meds Development Team   Jun. 1999
   Hypertension Development Team   Aug. 2002
   Supply chain (purchasing, recalls, etc.)
   Billing

Neuromusculoskeletal
   Total hip arthroplasty
   Total knee arthroplasty
   Low back pain
   Physical therapy

Surgical Specialties
   Pain Services Development Team   Sep. 2006
   General Surgery Development Team   Jan. 2007
   Surgical Support Services Development Team   Feb. 2007

Women & Newborns
   OB Development Team
      Elective induction (emergency C-section rates)
      Delivery-associated maternal injuries
      Neonatal bilirubin testing and treatment
   NICU Development Team
   Dysfunctional Uterine Bleeding Development Team

Intensive Medicine
   Critical Care Development Team   Mar. 2003
      Medical evaluation teams (RRTs)
      Central line sepsis
      Ventilator-associated pneumonia
      Blood glucose control
   Trauma Development Team   Apr. 2004
      Traumatic brain injury
   Emergency Care Development Team   Nov. 2004
      Febrile Infant
      AMI
      Sepsis

TABLE 7-1. (continued)
Intermountain Clinical Program and Development Teams*

Pneumonia	
Transport Development Team	Sep. 2004
Hospitalist Development Team	Feb. 2006
Inpatient pneumonia	
Inpatient DVT prevention and treatment	
Stroke Development Team	Jan. 2005

Intensive Pediatrics (started 2006—doing key process analysis)
Bronchiolitis

Intensive Behavioral (not yet started)

Oncology

Breast Cancer Development Team	May 2002
Breast-conserving treatment	
Axillary note dissection	
Sentinel node biopsy	
Mammography Development Team	Aug. 2004
Prostate Cancer Development Team	Mar. 2005
Neuro-oncology Development Team	Mar. 2005
Medical Oncology Development Team	Aug. 2005
Radiation Therapy Development Team	Mar. 2004

Primary Care

Community Health & Prevention Development Team	Jan. 1999
Preventive Care Guidelines and Tools	
(child, adolescent, adult; general disease screening)	
Immunizations	
(child, adolescent, adult, employee, pandemic planning)	
Obesity	
(adult, child, and adolescent)	
Tobacco	
Nutrition and activity	
Asthma Development Team	Jul. 1999
Diabetes Development Team	Jan. 1999
Lower Respiratory Infection Development Team	Jan. 2000
Community-acquired pneumonia	
Antibiotic use in bronchitis	
Otitis Media/Pediatric Respiratory Development Team	
Chronic Anticoagulation Development Team	Apr. 2001
Mental Health Integration Development Team	Jan. 1999
Depression	

* Start-up dates and individual Care Process Models (CPMs) are individually listed. When a development team (e.g., CV Surgery) has more than one CPM, or when the main CPM is not obvious from the development team's title, further notations are provided. IHD, ischemic heart disease; AMI, acute myocardial infarction; CHF, congestive heart failure; CV, cardiovascular; OB, obstetrics; C-section, Cesarean section; NICU, neonatal intensive care unit; RRTs, rapid response teams; DVT, deep vein thrombosis.

who see diabetes patients in their practices every day. The knowledge experts are diabetologists, drawn from each region.

A new development team begins its work by generating a CPM for its assigned key clinical process. Intermountain's central clinical program staff provide a great deal of coordinated support for this effort. A CPM development process contains five sequential elements:

1. The knowledge experts generate an evidence-based, best-practice guideline for the condition under study, with appropriate links to the published literature. They share their work with the development team, which in turn shares it with their frontline colleagues, asking, "What would you change?" Through iterations of mutual feedback and refinement, the shared baseline practice guideline stabilizes over time.

2. The full development team converts the practice guideline into clinical work flow documents suitable for use in direct patient care. This step is often the most difficult in the CPM development process. Good clinical flow can enhance clinical productivity, rather than adding burden to frontline practitioners. The aim is to make evidence-based best care the lowest-energy default option, with data collection integrated into clinical work flow.

   The core of most chronic disease CPMs is a "treatment cascade." Treatment cascades start with disease detection and diagnosis. The first (and most important) "treatment" is intensive patient education, enabling the patient to become the primary disease manager. The cascade then steps sequentially through increasing levels of treatment. A frontline clinical team moves down the cascade until it achieves adequate control of the patient's condition, while modifying the cascade's shared baseline as dictated by individual patient's needs. The last step in most cascades is referral to a specialist.

3. The team next applies the NQF outcomes tracking system development tools, producing a balanced dashboard of clinical, cost, and satisfaction outcomes. (*See* Sidebar 7-4, page 100, for discussion of balanced outcomes measurement.) This effort involves the electronic data warehouse team, which designs clinical registries that bring together complementary data flows with appropriate preprocessing.

4. The development team works with Intermountain's medical informatics groups to blend clinical work flow tools and data system needs into automated patient care data systems.

5. Central support staff help the development team build Web-based educational materials for both care delivery professionals and the patients they serve.

A finished CPM is formally deployed into clinical practice by the governing guidance council, through its regional physician/nurse leader dyads. The development team's role changes at that point. The team continues to meet monthly to review and update the CPM. The team's knowledge experts have funded time to track new research developments. The team also reviews care variations as clinicians adapt the shared baseline. It closely follows major clinical outcomes and receives and clears improvement ideas that arise among Intermountain's frontline practitioners and leaders.

As a result of this dynamic structure, Intermountain's CPMs tend to change quite frequently. Knowledge experts have an additional responsibility to share new findings and changes with their frontline colleagues. They conduct regular continuing education sessions, targeted at both practicing physicians and nonphysician staff. (Technically, this is called "academic detailing;" it is one of the few continuing education methods demonstrated to change clinical practice). Education sessions cover the full spectrum of the coordinated CPM. They review current best practice (the core evidence-based guideline), relate it to clinical work flow, show delivery teams how to track patient results through the outcomes data system, tie the CPM to decision support tools built into the electronic medical record, and link it to a full set of educational materials for patients and care delivery professionals.

Chronic disease knowledge experts also run the specialty clinics that support frontline care delivery teams. Continuing education sessions usually coordinate the logistics of that support. Finally, the knowledge experts coordinate specialty-based nurse care managers and patient trainers.

A CPM in Action: Diabetes Mellitus

Through its health plan and outpatient clinics, Intermountain supports more than 20,000 patients diagnosed with diabetes mellitus. Among approximately 800 primary care physicians who manage diabetic patients, one-third are employed within the Intermountain Medical Group, whereas the remainder are community-based, independent physicians. All physicians and their care delivery teams—regardless of employment status—interact regularly with the Primary Care Clinical Program medical directors and clinical operations administrators. They have access to regular diabetes continuing education sessions. Three endocrinologists (one in each region) act as knowledge experts on the Diabetes Development Team. In addition to conducting diabetes training, the knowledge experts coordinate specialty nursing care management (diabetic educators) and supply most specialty services.

Each quarter, Intermountain sends a set of reports to every clinical team managing diabetic patients. The reports are generated from the Diabetes Data Mart (a patient registry) within Intermountain's electronic data warehouse. The packet includes a Diabetes Action List. The action list summarizes every diabetic patient in the team's practice, listing testing rates and levels of control for standard clinical quality indicators such as glycolated hemoglobin (HA1C), low-density lipoproteins, blood pressure, urinary protein, dilated retinal exams, and pedal sensory exams. The report flags any care defect, as reflected either in test frequency or level of control. Frontline teams review the lists, then either schedule flagged patients for office visits, or assign them to general care management nurses at the local clinic. Although Intermountain puts Diabetes Action Lists out every quarter, frontline teams can generate them on demand. Most teams do so every month (*See* again Sidebar 7-4, page 100, on outcomes measurement).

In addition to action lists, frontline teams can access patient-specific patient worksheets through Intermountain's Web-based Results Review system. Most practices integrate the worksheets into their work flow during chart preparation. The worksheet contains patient demographics, a list of all active medications, and a review of pertinent history and laboratory results focused around chronic conditions. For diabetic patients, it will include test dates and values for the last seven HA1Cs, low-density lipoproteins, blood pressures, urinary proteins, dilated retinal examinations, and pedal sensory examinations. A final section of the worksheet applies all pertinent treatment cascades, listing recommendations for immunizations, disease screening, and appropriate testing. It will flag out-of-control levels, with next-step treatment recommendations. (Technically, this section of the worksheet is a passive form of computerized physician order entry).

The standard quarterly report packet also contains sections comparing each clinical team's risk-adjusted performance with its peers. A fourth report tracks progress on

quality improvement goals and links them to financial incentives. Finally, a separate summary report goes to the team's clinical program medical director. In meeting with the frontline teams, the clinical program leadership dyad often shares methods used by other practices to improve patient outcome performance, with specific practice flow recommendations (true benchmarking when combined with the peer comparison reports). Figures 7-2 (page 106) and 7-3 (page 107) show system-level performance on representative diabetes outcomes measures, as pulled in real time from the Intermountain outcomes tracking system. Primary care physicians supply almost 90% of all diabetes care in the system. As the last step in the diabetes treatment cascade, Intermountain's diabetes knowledge experts tend to concentrate the most difficult patients in their specialty practices. As a result, they typically have worse outcomes than their primary care colleagues.

Discussion and Conclusion
Using Routine Care Delivery to Generate Reliable Clinical Knowledge

Evidence-based best practice faces a massive evidence gap. The healing professions currently have reliable evidence (Level I, II, or III randomized trials, robust observational designs, or expert consensus opinion using formal methods)[14] to identify the best patient-specific practice for only a small minority of care delivery choices.[15] Bridging this gap will strain the capacity of any conceivable research system.

Intermountain designed its clinical programs to rationalize, optimize, and improve care delivery performance. The resulting organizational and information structures make it possible to generate robust data regarding treatment effects as a by-product of demonstrated best care. In this context, CPMs have several major virtues. They do the following:

- Embed data systems that directly link outcome results to care delivery decisions
- Deploy organized care delivery processes throughout the system
- Function as effectiveness "research engines" that are built systemwide into frontline care delivery

At a minimum, CPMs routinely generate Level II information (robust, prospective observational time series) for all key clinical care delivery processes. Because frontline care is supported by, and in turn supports, a data-rich and protocol-friendly infrastructure, all clinical care changes get tested. Changes such as newly published

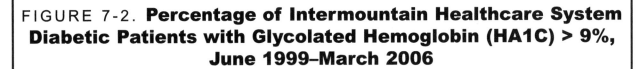

FIGURE 7-2. **Percentage of Intermountain Healthcare System Diabetic Patients with Glycolated Hemoglobin (HA1C) > 9%, June 1999–March 2006**

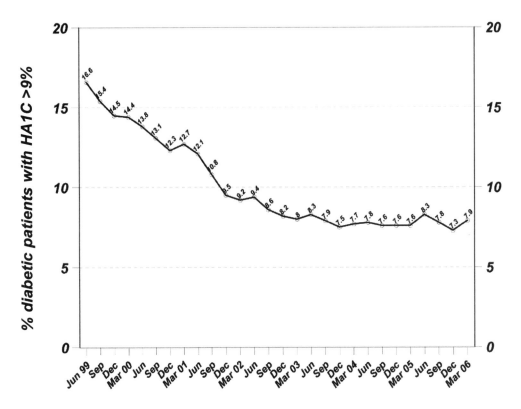

Figure 7-2. This figure represents data for more than 20,000 patients. National guidelines recommend that all patients with diabetes be managed to HA1C levels < 9%, and, ideally, to levels < 7%.

treatments in the medical literature, new medications, a new organizational structure for an intensive care unit, or a new nurse-staffing policy implementation, for example, can all generate robust information regarding their effectiveness.

As needed, development teams extend the scope of existing evidence as part of routine care delivery operations. For example,

- The Intermountain Cardiovascular Guidance Council developed robust observational evidence regarding discharge medications for patients hospitalized with ischemic heart disease or atrial fibrillation (Level II-2 evidence).[16]

- The Mental Health Integration Development Team used the Intermountain outcomes tracking system to conduct a prospective nonrandomized controlled trial (Level II-1 evidence) to assess the best practice for the detection and management of depression in primary care clinics.[17,18]

- The Lower Respiratory Infection Development Team ran a quasi-experiment that used existing prospective data flows to assess rollout of their community-acquired pneumonia (CAP) CPM (Level II-1 evidence).[19,20] This led to a randomized controlled trial to identify best antibiotic choices for outpatient management of CAP (Level I evidence).[21] With embedded data systems and an existing shared baseline care protocol that spanned the Intermountain system, the clinical trial was completed in less than three months. The largest associated expenses were Institutional Review Board oversight and data analysis—costs that Intermountain underwrote, based on a clear need to quickly generate and then to apply appropriate evidence to real patient care.

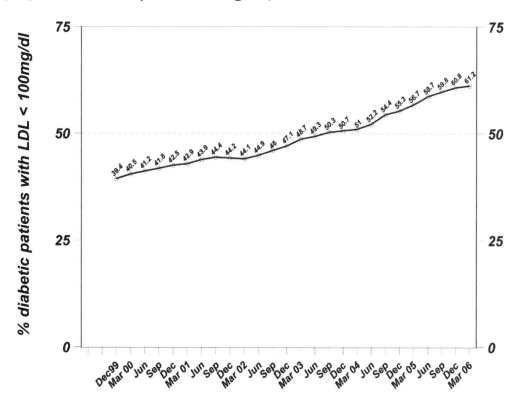

FIGURE 7-3. **Percentage of Intermountain Healthcare System Diabetic Patients with Lipid (Low-Density Lipoprotein/LDL) < 100 mg/dl, December 1999–March 2006**

Figure 7-3. This figure represents data for more than 20,000 patients. National guidelines recommend that all patients with diabetes be managed to LDL levels < 100 mg/dl.

Conclusion

By linking frontline (microsystem) care processes to organizational (mesosystem) information capacity and management infrastructure, Intermountain Healthcare enriches its quality improvement initiatives with quality control mechanisms that sustain improvements over time and that extend these improvements across an entire regional system of care. Such a program requires substantial organizational investment, but the returns on this investment are substantial as well. Patient outcomes are demonstrably improved, and service delivery is both effective and efficient. Clinicians feel supported in their provision of daily care and are motivated to engage in, and to sustain, the work of learning from practice and improving practice. Within Intermountain, when a physician says "in my experience," it means measured results, not individual anecdote in the form of a physi-

cian's subjective recall across patient groups over time (a practice with well-known significant limitations). In addition, by embedding effectiveness research within routine care processes, the organization can generate and rapidly deploy new clinical knowledge. Improvements in patient outcome, system performance, and practice-based research thus support each other, promoting best care for each patient "here in the room," while generating evidence on best care for patients in general.

References

1. Deming W.E.: *Out of the Crisis.* Cambridge, MA: Massachusetts Institute of Technology Center for Advanced Engineering Study, 1986.
2. Juran J.M., Gryna F.M. (eds.): *Juran's Quality Control Handbook,* 4th ed. New York City: McGraw-Hill, Inc., 1951.
3. Intermountain Healthcare: *About Intermountain: Serving Our Communities.* http://intermountainhealthcare.org/xp/public/aboutihc/ (accessed May 25, 2007).

4. Classen D.C., et al.: The timing of prophylactic administration of antibiotics and the risk of surgical wound infection. *N Engl J Med* 326:281–286, Jan. 30, 1992.

5. James B.C.: *Quality Management for Health Care Delivery* (monograph). Chicago: Hospital Research and Educational Trust (American Hospital Association), 1989.

6. James B.C.: Quality improvement opportunities in health care: Making it easy to do it right. *J Manag Care Pharm* 8:394–399, Sep./Oct. 2002.

7. James B.C.: Making it easy to do it right [editorial]. *N Engl J Med* 345:991–993, Sep. 27, 2001.

8. Institute of Medicine: *Crossing the Quality Chasm: A New Health System for the 21st Century.* Washington, DC: National Academy Press, 2001.

9. Batalden P., Splaine M.: What will it take to lead the continual improvement and innovation of health care in the 21st century? *Qual Manag Health Care* 11:45–54, Fall 2002.

10. Nelson E.C., et al.: Microsystems in health care: Part 1. Learning from high-performing front-line clinical units. *Jt Comm J Qual Improv* 28:472–493, Sep. 2002.

11. James B.C.: Information system concepts for quality measurement. *Med Care* 41:171–178, Jan. 2003.

12. Berwick D.M., James B.C., Coye M.J.: The connections between quality measurement and improvement. *Med Care* 41:130–139, Jan. 2003.

13. Casalino L.P.: The unintended consequences of measuring quality on the quality of medical care. *N Engl J Med* 341:1147–1150, Oct. 7, 1999.

14. Lawrence R., Mickalide A.: Preventive services in clinical practice: Designing the periodic health examination. *JAMA* 257:2205–2207, Apr. 24, 1987.

15. Williamson J., et al.: *Medical Practice Information Demonstration Project: Final Report.* Baltimore: Office of the Assistant Secretary of Health, Department of Health, Education, & Welfare, Contract #282-77-0068GS, Policy Research Inc., 1979.

16. Lappe J.M., et al. Improvements in 1-year cardiovascular clinical outcomes associated with a hospital-based discharge medication program. *Ann Intern Med* 141:446–453, Sep. 21, 2004.

17. Reiss-Brennan B., et al.: Mental health integration: Rethinking practitioner roles in the treatment of depression: The specialist, primary care physicians, and the practice nurse. *Ethn Dis* 16(Suppl 3):S3-37–S3-43, Spring 2006.

19. Dean N., Bateman K.: Local guidelines for community-acquired pneumonia: Development, implementation, and outcome studies. *Infect Dis Clin North Am* 18:975–991, Dec. 2004.

20. Dean N.C., et al.: Decreased mortality after implementation of a treatment guideline for community-acquired pneumonia. *Am J Med* 110:451–457, Apr. 15, 2001.

21. Dean N.C., et al.: Improved clinical outcomes with utilization of a community-acquired pneumonia guideline. *Chest* 130:794–799, Sep. 2006.

Developing Improvement Skills in Clinician Learners: Defining the Core Competencies of Physicians

Tina C. Foster, Greg S. Ogrinc

What I hear, I forget. What I see, I remember. What I do, I understand. —Confucius[1]

As members of the inpatient team complete morning rounds, they return to the conference room to discuss patients on their hospital services. The attending physician asks for an update on the glucose control of the team's diabetic patients. Andy, the third-year medical student, pulls out a summary sheet he prepared after reviewing relevant articles from the medical literature. He reports that morbidity and mortality are decreased in hospitalized patients whose blood sugars are maintained between 80 and 180.[2] Adam, the intern, then summarizes the prior 24 hours of blood sugars for diabetic patients on the service. Three of the four patients have had more than 75% of their blood glucose readings in the target range. The attending physician updates a chart on the white board that tracks progress the team is making. One patient's readings have been persistently greater than 200. This is concerning for the team, so Leslie, the fourth-year pharmacy student, and Andy get together to revise the treatment regimen for this patient. Leslie and Andy review the recommendations from the literature, check the medication formulary at the hospital, then finalize the plan with Annette, the supervising resident on the team. Annette suggests discussing the plan with the patient's nurse to ensure that the recommendation is congruent with nursing work load on the ward.

As the above case example makes clear, the activities of patient care, practice improvement, and professional learning are interdependent and mutually supportive. Clinician-learners from many disciplines can work together on these tasks during usual rounds, so that practice-based learning and improvement (PBLI) are not additions to a busy day but rather integral components. For this type of integrated education to be effective, however, health professionals at all levels of experience must recognize opportunities for improvement-based learning, and must master skills to act on these opportunities when they arise.

The current chapter explores PBLI from a developmental perspective. We ask how improvement-oriented educational experiences can be built into different stages of professional training and how these experiences can be tailored to the evolving needs and capacities of clinician-learners. In addition, we consider the efforts of accrediting organizations to support development of health professionals who are competent in the continual improvement of care as a usual component of delivering care.

Defining Core Competency

Quality improvement (QI) is an increasingly visible aspect of clinical practice, but such work will not become normative until training in essential improvement skills is built into every level of health professional preparation. Fortunately, major educational and accrediting organizations have begun to recognize this requirement. The American Association of Colleges of Nursing and the American Nursing Association[3] have endorsed quality improvement as a core element of nurse education. The Accreditation Council for Pharmacy Education[4] incorporates knowledge and skills for medication safety, QI, and work in interdisciplinary teams as part of its standards for pharmacy students. Physician training has incorporated QIon two fronts: (1) the Association of American Medical Colleges (AAMC) has recommended goals related to QI for medical students[5] and (2) the Accreditation Council for Graduate Medical Education (ACGME) includes PBLI and systems-based practice as two of six core competencies for all resident physicians trained in the United States.[6]

In many ways, ACGME has led the charge for practice-based learning and improvement training. In the late 1990s, the ACGME Outcome Project identified four main goals:

1. Define general competencies for residency training.
2. Support programs in assessing these competencies.
3. Develop models of dependable resident evaluation systems.
4. Create resources and support systems for resident physician programs.

Goal 1 specifies six essential competencies: medical knowledge, patient care, interpersonal communication, professionalism, system-based practice, and PBLI. Goals 2–4 provide ongoing support to residency programs. In our consideration of PBLI as a core clinical competency, we must reflect on the term *competency* itself, as it was chosen for a specific reason. Why not choose six "skills" to master? Or six "domains of learning?"

The term *competency* was chosen because it links stages of professional development with general models of adult learning. Although different individuals acquire and assimilate knowledge and skills in different ways, an appreciation of general developmental stages permits both learners and educators (including instructors, mentors, and coaches) to create and structure optimal learning experiences. ACGME adapted a model developed by Hubert and Stewart Dreyfus in the 1970s.[7] Focusing on chess players and pilots, the Dreyfus brothers described five stages (and characteristics) of skill development: novice, advanced beginner, competent, proficient, and expert (Table 8-1, page 111). Because it is ACGME's expectation that resident physicians achieve a level of competence by the end of training, clinical educators must understand the experience of learners in each of the Dreyfus stages:[8]

1. **Novice.** At the novice level, learners attend to basic rules themselves rather than to real-world application of these rules. (In the spirit of Dragnet, novices want "just the facts.") Instructors, in turn, must make these rules the focus of their educational efforts. Knowledge at this level is free of context, and as a result, learners' application of such rules might produce poor results in the real world. For example, the medical student

will learn the four locations of stethoscope placement for cardiac auscultation.

2. **Advanced Beginner.** As the novice gains initial experience with real situations, he or she progresses to the next level. Experience interacts with and contextualizes the rule itself, and the nature of the interaction becomes important. This work in context enhances the basic knowledge. In our example of cardiac auscultation, the medical student begins to experience heart sounds with many patients in various clinical contexts (a healthy pregnant woman, a newborn baby, a well child exam, or a patient with symptoms of heart disease).

3. **Competent.** As the advanced beginner gains further experience, the number and variation of elements in the situation can become overwhelming. Learners begin to appreciate, however, which elements of the situation require attention and which do not. The vast possibilities (of interpretation or action) can be narrowed to a manageable few. In addition, a deep emotional attachment to the task now develops. The successes, failures, joys, and disappointments matter on a much deeper level. To continue our example, a medical student is able to recognize abnormal heart sounds in patients for whom an abnormal finding is expected (for example, a blue baby, a middle-aged man with known valvular disease, or an easily fatigued older woman).

4. **Proficient.** This is an extension of the level of competence. The learner continues to scroll through a complete list of possibilities but does so with much greater speed. An element of efficiency now accompanies the proficiency. Individuals develop the capacity to step back and see more clearly the problem that needs to be solved, although often the solution itself still requires active deliberation. Increased efficiency enables the practitioner to remove waste from the work by directly connecting knowledge and skill to the problem at hand. For example, a resident physician might recognize that a patient is sick and realize that the differential diagnosis is large. However, he moves quickly and discovers a new systolic murmur over the aortic valve. This rules out many possibilities and enables working expeditiously through the differential diagnosis.

5. **Expert.** The expert develops a vast repertoire of skills and a capacity for situational discrimination that are only achievable through experience. Tasks are per-

formed on a more intuitive level, and essential problems are recognized and immediately addressed. Expert practitioners also learn to comfortably manage situations in which the rules do not apply. So, to complete our example, the expert intuitively integrates the status of a murmur in an otherwise healthy person, rapidly identifies the issues that could be problematic if ignored, and focuses work directly on these concerns.

In adapting the developmental language of the Dreyfus model to the specific challenges of health professional training, ACGME has recognized that this training is a process of ongoing growth and development. Acquisition of specific knowledge and skills is essential for all professionals, but terms such as *competent* and *proficient* direct our attention to practitioners' underlying capacity to assimilate and *apply* this knowledge and these

skills with increasing sophistication in the work of health care. As today's competent medical resident matures into tomorrow's proficient and expert practitioner, PBLI must mature and develop along with clinical knowledge and clinical decision-making skills do.

Developing Competency in Practice-Based Learning and Improvement

As has been emphasized throughout this book, health care improvement is not a "spectator sport" but a participant-driven implementation of specific knowledge and skills. It cannot be learned passively by sitting in a lecture, watching a DVD, attending a meeting, or visiting Web sites, although Web sites, didactic sessions, and other materials can play an important role in preparing the learner. Improvement is an action and its learning must be action-

TABLE 8-1. Dreyfus Levels of Skill Development*

Learner Level	Characteristics and Behaviors
Novice	• Uses the basic rules and "rules of thumb" • Context free • Rules are applied only using the basic features
Advanced Beginner	• Begins to gain experience in the real world • Develops context for the tasks and the context adds new information to the task
Competent	• Can differentiate which elements of the situation are important to attend to and which are not • Can restrict to only a few of the vast possibilities • Develops an emotional attachment to the task
Proficient	• Continues to scroll through all the possibilities, but does so with greater speed • Takes waste out of the tasks/work • Can step back and see the problem that needs to be solved
Expert	• Has developed a vast repertoire of situational discrimination that is only achievable through experience • Works intuitively on the problem • Is comfortable working where the rules do not apply

* Note: *See* text for health care example of clinical skill development.

based as well. But what skills and knowledge are required at each stage in this learning process, so that students and residents achieve competence in PBLI before entering practice as health care professionals? Let us more closely examine each stage in this professional development so that we can identify specific improvement-oriented educational strategies.

Initiating the Novice

Health professional students begin their training as novices of PBLI, and they benefit from exposure to generic "rules" of improvement. The Institute for Healthcare Improvement (IHI) has identified eight domains of knowledge for improvement work (Table 8-2, page 113).[9] These domains serve as a valuable framework for introducing students to PBLI theory and practice and for fostering PBLI curriculum development among faculty. Of course, even this framework (which we have found to be quite useful) might feel abstract to the novice with minimal real-world experience. A bridge to such experience, in contexts familiar to the student, can bring improvement principles to life.

One means of achieving this bridge is through a *personal improvement project*. The learner is invited to define an aim, to describe measures, to collect data, and to complete one or more plan-do-study-act cycles that improve performance in a domain of personal relevance. Novice practitioners of improvement (and experienced practitioners as well) can address a range of issues, from the personal (diet, exercise, housework) to the professional (study habits, time management, experience with clinical preceptors). Students enjoy the opportunity to apply new knowledge in a safe environment. In this context they gain comfort and facility with more widely applicable improvement techniques. Experience with nursing students has shown personal improvement projects to be an effective way to introduce the principles above.[10]

Students also bring naïve eyes to the study of health care processes, and their perspective is valuable to improvement teams that seek to describe existing health care processes. Involving students in specific aspects of improvement work enables them to contribute insights that might be missed by more senior clinicians who are immersed everyday in the (dys)functions of the health care system.

Developing Advanced Beginner Knowledge and Skills

The advanced beginner needs many opportunities to apply rules in action. Such opportunities can be construct-

ed around formal PBLI rotations or other hands-on experiences. These contexts also enable students to participate in (and to reap the benefits of) interdisciplinary learning, specifically through collaboration with learners in other disciplines such as nursing, pharmacy, and health administration. Many professional schools and postgraduate education programs have developed integrated experiences that allow learners to simultaneously learn about PBLI and to improve patient care at the front line.

In some cases linking learners with an existing improvement initiative is helpful, but challenges can arise related to project duration, schedule conflicts, and perceived relevance (to the student's particular goals and interests). Alternatively, allowing learners themselves to identify an area for improvement, and then pairing them with a mentor to design and execute a project of appropriate scope, can be a very successful strategy. Learners at the advanced beginner level can apply theories and basic skills they learned as novices, and can experience what happens when theory bumps into reality. They also deeply value the opportunity to contribute to visible improvement in patient care.

Since 2003, all second-year medical students at the University Of Minnesota School of Medicine have completed a Health Improvement Project as part of Physician and Society, the second year introduction to clinical medicine course. After learning the basics of PBLI in their first year, these students work together in groups of 8 to 12 individuals; each group works with a project site in the Twin Cities community. Students are invited to evaluate the gap between actual and ideal care outcomes, and then to develop strategies that close this gap. "Products" from student projects have included a pamphlet on peripheral vascular disease for Native American women, improved reproductive health teaching for Hispanic youth, and development of a video to teach health care professionals about rapid response teams. These are but a few examples of students' successful efforts to identify a health care gap and to take the initial steps toward closure of that gap and improve care for patients, all in a context that supports professional development of the learners themselves.

Competence and Beyond

Developing competence (and proficiency or expertise) in PBLI is essential not only for students but also for practicing professionals. Practicing physicians will soon be expected to demonstrate competence in PBLI as part of their Maintenance of Certification. The American Board of Medical Specialties defines four components required

TABLE 8-2. Institute for Healthcare Improvement (IHI) Eight Knowledge Domains for the Improvement of Health Care

1. Customer/beneficiary knowledge	• Identification of the person, persons, or groups for whom health care is provided • Assessment of their needs and preferences • The relationship of the health care provided to those needs and preferences
2. Health care as process, system	• The interdependent people (patients, families, eligible populations, caregivers), procedures, activities, and technologies of health care–giving that come together to meet the need(s) of individuals and communities
3. Variation and measurement	• The use of measurement to understand the variation of performance in processes and systems of work • Used to improve the design and redesign of health care
4. Leading, following, and making changes in health care	• The methods and skills for making change in complex organizations • The general and strategic management of people and the health care work they do (financing, information technology, daily health care–giving)
5. Collaboration	• The knowledge, methods, and skills needed to work effectively in groups • The understanding and valuing of the perspectives and responsibilities of others • The capacity to foster the same in others
6. Developing new, locally useful knowledge	• The recognition of the need for new knowledge in personal daily health professional practice • The skill to develop new knowledge through empiric testing
7. Social context and accountability	• An understanding of the social contexts (local, regional, national, global) of health care • The financial impact and costs of health care
8. Professional subject matter	• The health professional knowledge appropriate for a specific discipline • The ability to apply and connect it to all of the above • Core competencies published by professional boards, accrediting organizations, and other certifying entities

Source: Institute for Healthcare Improvement: *Eight Knowledge Domains for Health Professional Students.* http://www.ihi.org/IHI/Topics/HealthProfessionsEducation/EducationGeneral/EmergingContent/EightKnowledge DomainsforHealthProfessionalStudents.htm (accessed May 31, 2007). Used with permission.

for Maintenance of Certification, one of which is "Practice Performance Assessment." Physicians in all member specialties will be asked to demonstrate that they can assess the quality of care they provide compared to peers and national benchmarks and then apply the best evidence or consensus recommendations to improve that care using follow-up assessments.[11] Because most residency programs (like most undergraduate health professional education programs) provide only introductory knowledge and experience with improvement methods, adequate preparation for competent practitioners can be challenging to achieve. Faculty who are skilled and comfortable teaching PBLI are still relatively limited in number. Many also have significant competing demands on their time.

Although existing institutional infrastructure is often inadequate to support effective teaching (and practice) of PBLI, some programs have significantly redesigned their own teaching and practice structures, and have developed specific learning experiences to prepare competent PBLI practitioners. The AAMC Chronic Care Collaborative, for example, has been very successful in coordinating patient care and practice redesign with formal PBLI teaching. This collaboration across more than 20 medical centers has resulted in many resident practices outperforming staff physician practices in outcomes for diabetes care. As emphasized previously, the activities of patient care, practice improvement, and professional learning are interdependent and mutually supportive, especially when thoughtful planning supports the integration.

In another example, the Dartmouth-Hitchcock Leadership Preventive Medicine Residency program offers a new approach to preventive medicine training, linking it with the other clinical residencies offered at the institution and requiring a major leadership experience in PBLI for successful program completion. Program residents have redesigned care for patients with community-acquired pneumonia, improved care for diabetics in both the hospital and the outpatient setting, increased the safety and efficacy of sedation for endoscopic procedures, and optimized use of electronic medical records to address obesity in a community health clinic. In this work, residents find themselves working closely with the many individuals who provide care for a given population of patients. This gives them new insight into the professional roles and activities of a wide variety of health professionals. Collaboration takes on a new meaning when it is focused around understanding the process of care for a group of patients; residents discover interdependencies of which

they were previously unaware, and they develop a real appreciation for the skills that nonphysicians bring to the enterprise. As residents move beyond a training model that is focused on a series of individual patient encounters, they come to recognize the complexity of the systems in which they work. They also develop a much deeper understanding of what is needed to make change in their workplace.

This leadership experience occupies two full years of residency, with the first year being devoted primarily to understanding the health care processes and outcomes for a population of patients treated at the medical center, and the second year devoted to a leaders practicum experience in which residents lead change for the improvement of those patients' care. All practicums are approved by a review board that includes senior leaders of the institution. The program benefits from extensive coordination between academic and clinical settings, and enjoys significant support from senior leaders of the institution. Such commitment is possible because the program not only develops knowledge and skills in both residents and faculty, but also stimulates tangible improvements in patient experience and outcomes, with anticipated health system cost reductions as well.

Educational Programs' Self-Improvement

In July 2006, the ACGME Outcome Project moved into its third phase, requiring graduate medical education (GME) programs to demonstrate their use of resident outcomes for program improvement. Such demonstration requires that programs know the needs of the population they are training, understand their own training processes and patterns, define measures related to educational outcomes, collect data on those outcomes, and develop ways to improve the training processes, all of which should result in improved outcomes. In other words, residency program directors must use PBLI knowledge and skills on their own programs! Although this mandate represents a challenge to program directors, who must endeavor to learn more about their own educational processes and outcomes (including patient care outcomes), it also provides both faculty and residents with new opportunities to teach and to learn the methods of PBLI.

Learning portfolios are one way to record and to reflect on experiences, an essential aspect of PBLI. An extensive literature exists on the use of learning portfolios in health professional education and on their value to students and practicing professionals.[12-14] With the increased emphasis on documentation of learner progress and development of reflective learning skills, the use of portfolios in health professional education is increasing. One example is activity underway at the ACGME. Seeing the potential benefit to residents, residency programs, and the accreditation process, the ACGME is moving forward with development of a portfolio system. Such a portfolio not only will help residents to better understand their own experience and progress in training but can serve as the basis for a lifelong portfolio that is maintained after the completion of residency. Program directors will have better information about their residents' learning, and can use these aggregated outcomes for program improvements. An institution can use aggregated outcomes across programs to improve its GME offerings. Finally, accreditors will have the ability to look at aggregated outcomes as they evaluate programs. Portfolio users will be able to share evaluation tools and best practices, developing a community around portfolio use and educational improvement.

As the health care systems evolves, our current health professional students will become the leaders of tomorrow: clinicians, administrators, and researchers. PBLI is a core competency that all must achieve. Starting early in training will ensure the strongest foundation so that the knowledge and skills of improvement are woven into the fabric of their professional activity. We are excited by the transformative potential of this work. Developing a community of learners around educational PBLI will strengthen interdisciplinary collaboration, promote professional development, and improve both the processes and outcomes of patient care.

References

1. Quote DB. http://www.quotedb.com/quotes/1492 (accessed Jun. 25, 2007).
2. Van den Berghe G. Insulin therapy for the critically ill patient. *Clin Cornerstone* 5(2):56–63, 2004.
3. Cronenwett L., et al.: Quality and safety education for nurses. *Nurs Outlook* 55:122–131, May–Jun. 2007.
4. Accreditation Council for Pharmacy Education: *Accreditation Standards and Guidelines.* http://www.acpe-accredit.org/standards/default.asp (accessed May 31, 2007).
5. Batalden P.: *Report V: Contemporary Issues in Medicine: Quality of Care.* Washington DC: Association of American Medical Colleges, Aug. 2001.
6. Leach D.C.: Evaluation of competency: An ACGME perspective. Accreditation Council for Graduate Medical Education. *Am J Phys Med Rehabil* 79:487–489, Sep.–Oct. 2000.
7. Dreyfus H., Dreyfus S.: *Mind Over Medicine.* New York City: Free Press, 1982.
8. Ogrinc G., et al.: A framework for teaching medical students and residents about practice-based learning and improvement, synthesized from the literature. *Acad Med* 78:748–756, Jul. 2003.
9. Institute for Healthcare Improvement: *Eight Knowledge Domains for Health Professional Students.* http://www.ihi.org/IHI/Topics/HealthProfessionsEducation/EducationGeneral/EmergingContent/EightKnowledgeDomainsforHealthProfessionalStudents.htm (accessed May 31, 2007).
10. Kyrkjebo J.M., Hanestad B.R.: Personal improvement project in nursing education: Learning methods and tools for continuous quality improvement in nursing practice. *J Adv Nurs* 41:88–98, Jan. 2003.
11. American Board of Medical Specialties: *Maintenance of Certification (MOC).* http://www.abms.org/About_Board_Certification/MOC.aspx (accessed May 31, 2007).
12. Carraccio C., Englander R.: Evaluating competence using a portfolio: A literature review and Web-based application to the ACGME competencies. *Teach Learn Med* 16:381–387, Fall 2004.
13. Challis M.: AMEE Medical Education Guide no. 11 (revised): Portfolio-based learning and assessment in medical education. *Med Teach* 21:370–386, Jul. 1999.
14. McMullan M., et al.: Portfolios and assessment of competence: A review of the literature. *J Adv Nurs* 41:283–294, Feb. 2003.

Applying the Idea: Advanced Applications of Clinical Value Compass Thinking in Practice-Based Learning and Improvement

Eugene C. Nelson, Paul B. Batalden, Joel S. Lazar, James D. Weinstein, William H. Edwards

"Start with the ground you know, the pale ground beneath your feet…Start right now, take a small step you can call your own."
—David Whyte[1]

Our first steps toward clinical improvement might indeed feel like small ones, as the task before us is so great. In a system so vast and complex as modern medicine, we might struggle to imagine how small tests of local change can meaningfully alter outcomes beyond our practice's front door. But larger changes are indeed built up from mutually supportive smaller ones, and improvement methods appropriate to microsystem levels of care can be effectively applied at the mesosystem and macrosystem levels as well.

This final chapter presents advanced applications of improvement thinking in general and of Clinical Value Compass principles in particular, as developed in increasingly complex and inclusive systems of care. We review several case studies that illustrate the forms of knowledge and action we have previously explored, in contexts that extend local implementation to regional, national, and even global domains.

Chapters 4 and 7 emphasized the building of value compass–based data collection into daily work routines; in the present chapter this same principle drives Dartmouth Spine Center's leadership of a multicenter clinical trial. Chapter 5 reviewed important benchmarking techniques that facilitate the identification and sharing of best clinical practices, and this theme reappears in our description below of the Vermont Oxford Network (VON) of Intensive Care Nurseries (ICNs). Chapters 2, 3, and 6 underscored the role of all health care professionals in defining top priorities for change. Our discussion of the Institute for Healthcare Improvement demonstrates the implementation of this philosophy at a national level. Chapter 8 (and other chapters) underlined the importance of aligning improvement initiatives with clinicians' own continuous learning. Throughout the current chapter we again recognize the hands-on learning that proceeds in parallel with health care improvement—and that indeed directs and refines this work.

Our goal in this final chapter is to "start close in" (as the poet David Whyte reminds us), to "start with the ground [we] know," and to see how far our steps can carry us.

Case 1. The Dartmouth Spine Center's Use of Clinical Value Compass Thinking for Individual Patients, Clinical Improvement, and Clinical Research

Background: The Need for Innovation

One of us [J.D.W.] had a dream in the mid-1990s to develop a world-class program that would excel in the provision of care to patients with back pain and related disorders—getting people back to work and back to play, one back at a time—while supporting sophisticated research to advance orthopedic knowledge and clinical practice. The Dartmouth Spine Center was opened in 1996 as a major step toward realization of this dream.

To achieve "best performance" in both clinical outcomes and clinical service delivery, a patient-based information system was required that could capture and coordinate relevant data in real time and across multiple outcome domains. Such an "ideal" system would integrate and longitudinally display the following:

- Data from patients—self-reported information on health and functional status, expectations for care, and satisfaction with outcomes of care

- Data from providers—clinician-reported information on signs, symptoms, morbidities, assessments, diagnoses, and treatments
- Data from clinical and administrative sources—test results and billing information

Unfortunately, no such information system existed in 1996. A first imperative for the Spine Center was thus to develop such capacity, and to this end the Clinical Value Compass was a powerful tool.

Clinical Setting: Location of the Work

Located at Dartmouth-Hitchcock Medical Center (DHMC) in Lebanon, New Hampshire, the Spine Center supports a multidisciplinary staff committed not only to clinical care for patients with back and neck problems but also to patient-oriented research and to pre- and postgraduate education for health professionals. The Center leads large-scale clinical research programs funded by the National Institutes of Health, and it participates in the National Spine Center Network (established in 1994),

sharing comparative data with approximately 30 different clinical programs on treatment and outcomes for patients with spine disease.

Innovation: Novel Application of Clinical Value Compass Concepts

The Spine Center was among the first clinical programs to combine methods of "feed forward" and "feedback" data management to facilitate both patient care and system improvement. Rich streams of health information are generated in real time, available to the practitioner for point-of-care clinical service, and available (in aggregate) to the entire center for continuous monitoring and modifying of service delivery. Data collected early in the care episode are "fed forward" to both patient and provider during subsequent stages of the same and future encounters, supporting clinical decision-making and intervention. The same data are "fed back" to aggregated information systems to support local improvement and multi-institutional research.[2] Figure 9-1 (below) illustrates this important data streaming concept.

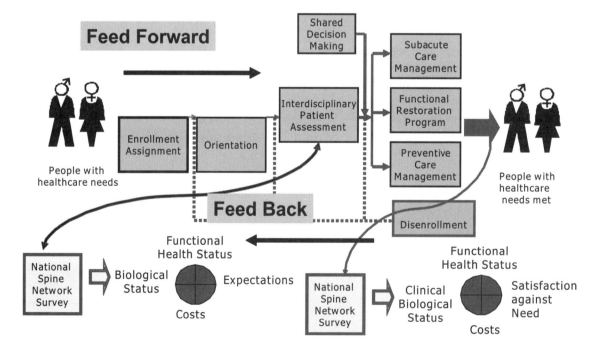

FIGURE 9-1. Feed-Forward and Feed-Back Data for Use in Patient Care, Program Improvement, and Clinical Research

Figure 9-1. Data collected early in the care episode are "fed forward" to both patient and provider during subsequent stages of the same and future encounters, supporting clinical decision making and intervention. The same data are "fed back" to aggregated information systems to support local improvement and multi-institutional research.

To achieve these simultaneous goals of patient care, program improvement, and clinical research, the Spine Center has built value compass thinking into every facet of its data management process, from collection to analysis to display. The Clinical Value Compass provides a master scheme for specifying required data elements and for planning flow of information during regular delivery of care.

Methods: How It Works

The Spine Center information system is patient-centered and multisourced. It combines encounter-specific survey data (collected via touch-pad technology at the time of the patient's Spine Center visit) with results from laboratory and radiology databases and with information from scheduling and billing sources that serve the entire DHMC.

When new patients present to the Spine Center, they are asked by the receptionist to complete a health assessment questionnaire on a laptop, touch-screen computer. Specific questions probe each Clinical Value Compass domain, with attention to general and spine-related health, functional and occupational status, expectations for specific treatment outcomes, satisfaction with care, and demographic background. Patients complete this assessment in 20 minutes, on average, and more than 95% of respondents can do so without assistance. Alternatively, some individuals choose to complete the survey at home, prior to their first appointment, using Internet-based software.

At the time of registration, each new patient completes a health survey, which is based on a survey developed by the National Spine Network, and the completed survey is uploaded to a central information system. The survey is scored instantly and automatically, and a one-page summary report, which includes a value compass–style printout unique to this patient, is generated in time for the actual clinician encounter.

Figure 9-2 (page 120) shows a sample summary sheet for a fictional but not atypical Spine Center patient making his second visit to the Spine Center. This 45-year-old, 270-pound white man has substantial back, buttock, and hip pain—the back pain has a long history. He has multiple comorbidities (hypertension, diabetes, stomach problem, and depression). He is unable to work full time and receives Social Security disability benefits. His functional status is poor; compared to national norms, he has low physical, emotional, and role function and may be clinically depressed at the time of the visit. He has had a variety of treatments during the past six months (for example, physical therapy, injections, massage, medications) from assorted clinicians but reports not only that he is not improving but that he is probably getting worse. He is currently taking anti-inflammatory and pain medications, which provide some symptom relief, although he believes that his back pain has worsened since his first visit to the Spine Center. He is dissatisfied with the degree of improvement he has achieved and with his treatment.

All this information, which is available at the beginning of the visit and is visible to both the patient and the clinician, can be used as a basis for assessment and for developing a shared plan of care that is most likely to meet the patient's needs and preferences. The patient has a discussion with the physician about his current state and the unsuccessful attempts to improve his health. The physician then tells the patient that many patients have benefited from a special, intensive program offered by the Spine Center, the Functional Restoration Program, which has been designed to help people improve their physical and mental health and regain their ability to work and to do the things they want to do. After learning more about the program by visiting the Center for Shared Decision Making, the patient meets with the Functional Restoration Program staff and decides to enter the program. His data will be tracked over time on the basis of the same metrics to determine if this new program is working for him.

As the above case example illustrates, when patients and practitioners meet, substantial data are available and organized in a manner that serves their mutual goal of value-focused care. The value compass–based patient summary directs clinicians' attention to patient-specific priorities and thus facilitates the process of shared decision making. It also highlights any "red flags" that warrant immediate attention or referral (for example, nocturnal symptoms that may require further diagnostic testing, suggestions of depression that may require psychology consultation).

Patient-based sources of data are subsequently merged with provider-based data, including standardized and templated information relevant to clinical findings, ordered treatments, and follow-up care plans. Laboratory, radiology, and billing information are incorporated as well. At subsequent visits, both patients and clinicians complete repeat assessments, and these data permit tracking of changes in health outcomes and perceptions over time, in response to specific therapeutic interventions.

Consequently, the Spine Center succeeds in generating a deep and longitudinal database on each patient, merging patient-based with provider-based information,

FIGURE 9-2. A Clinical Value Compass Display for an Individual Spine Center Patient

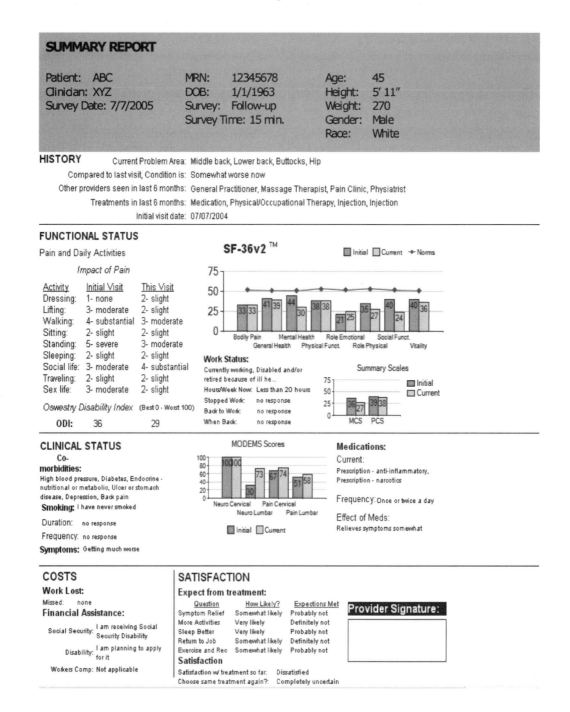

Figure 9-2. A Clinical Value Compass display for a second-time visitor to the Spine Center is shown. SF-36 refers to the self-administered SF-36® questionnaire. Reproduced with permission of Dynamic Clinical Systems, Inc., 2007. All rights reserved.

and combining problem-specific with general demographic information. These data continually evolve, informing clinical management in a "feed forward" manner. Simultaneously (as elaborated subsequently), information is aggregated across patients for "feedback" to local providers, and to the larger Spine Network, stimulating local improvement and collaborative research.

Displays and Utility: What It Looks Like and How It's Used

The fictional patient's Clinical Value Compass that is presented in Figure 9-2 (page 120) features a single-page format that displays (all in one viewing) clinical status, functional status, perceptions of treatment success, and other information such as occupational history and background. Functional status results (scores on a self-administered SF-36® questionnaire[3]) are mapped against a national sample of average adults. As time passes and as care progresses, changes in the value compass–based outcomes are measured quantitatively and are available for patient discussion, therapeutic monitoring (and adjustment), and aggregated performance assessment.

This aggregation of real-time data serves multiple goals. Figure 9-3 (page 122), for example, presents Clinical Value Compass data on a cohort of the Spine Center's patients with herniated disk. This information can be used by staff to set priorities for clinical program improvement and to monitor success of these improvements over time. For example, Spine Center staff at an annual retreat could look at these results and conclude that 70% of herniated disk patients had improved on the Oswestry Disability Index, which shows how pain affects daily activities, but that 33% still have pain at follow-up in the neck, back, or legs all or most of the time, and that only 50% improved on role functioning. The staff might decide to further investigate what they might do to decrease the rate of chronic pain at follow-up and to improve role functioning results.

The same information can be adapted to foster the Spine Center's expressed values of patient choice, shared decision making, and public transparency. Figure 9-4 (page 123), for example, depicts performance data as displayed on DHMC's publicly accessible Web site (http://www.DHMC.org). Because these data communicate honest and accurate information on relevant outcomes and costs, prospective patients are empowered to make more informed choices regarding their own clinical care. For example, if a patient had received a diagnosis of spinal stenosis (a common diagnosis among people suffering from low back pain), he or she could view the DHMC performance data and learn that treatment improved the condition of 25.5% of patients who chose nonsurgery care but 65.6% of patients who chose surgery. This could help the patient make a more informed decision about which path to chose and to have more information to use in making a good decision in consultation with his or her physician and family.

Finally, the Spine Center's "feed forward" data system connects to the National Spine Network database and facilitates large-scale clinical research. The value compass–based system has been adapted by and used in 13 other medical centers, in 11 states, as the informatics structure for a 15-million-dollar National Institutes of Health–sponsored randomized controlled trial on spinal surgery. Data from this trial have shed new light on the relative value of surgical versus nonsurgical interventions for common problems of the lower back.[4] Again, the Clinical Value Compass has guided investigators' identification, clarification, and longitudinal monitoring of outcome measures most important to patient care.

Case 2. The Vermont Oxford Network's Use of Clinical Value Compass Thinking for Learning and Benchmarking for Improvement

Background: The Need for Innovation

When another author (W.H.E.), as medical director of DHMC's intensive care nursery (ICN), was asked to define a vision for this clinical microsystem, another dream was articulated: "to achieve the best outcomes in the world." The means to such an end were not immediately apparent. Certainly, members of the ICN staff were talented and hardworking individuals and were committed to clinical excellence. But how could these professionals be effectively directed to achievement of "best-in-the-world" outcomes, and indeed, how might such outcomes even be identified? Two strategic interventions have proven especially valuable in this regard: alliance with the VON and implementation (both locally and internationally, in the context of this larger network) of value compass techniques.

Clinical Setting: Location of the Work

Established in 1988 by Drs. Jerold Lucey and Jeffrey Horbar and their North American and European colleagues, the VON is an international clinical association of more than 450 neonatal intensive care units (NICUs).

FIGURE 9-3. A Clinical Value Compass Display for a Cohort of Spine Center Patients with Herniated Disk

Spine Center's Surgical Herniated Disk Patients

Functional Health Status

Clinical Status

Common Health Problems	
Comorbidities besides spine condition	57%
Depression	18%
Frequent Headaches	18%
High Blood Pressure	14%
Osteoarthritis	11%
Heart Disease	5%

Symptoms	Initial	Followup	Improved
Oswestry Disability Index: How pain has affected your ability to perform activities	46	71	70%
MODEMS: Degree of suffering and bothersome			
Numbness, tingling, and/or weakness in *lower* body	41	70	69%
Numbness, tingling, and/or weakness in *upper* body	77	89	43%

Oswestry Disability Index (ODI): reported as low score is more disability
Improved for ODI is a difference of 10 points or greater between Followup and Initial
Improved for MODEMS is a difference of 5 points or greater between Followup and Initial

Pain at Followup	
Experience pain in the neck, arms, lower back, and/or legs most or all of the time	33%

Medications at Followup	
Taking medication(s)	61%

SF-36 Norm-based (mean 50 SD 10)	Initial	Followup	Improved
Bodily Pain	26	40	77%
Role Physical	27	37	50%
Physical Component Summary	28	38	62%
Mental Component Summary	43	51	58%
General Health			
Excellent & Very Good	40%	43%	26%

Improved for SF-36 is a difference of 5 points or greater between Followup and Initial
Improved for General Health is a positive change in category from Initial to Followup

Patient Case Mix (July '98 to Mar. '02)	
Patients (have followup survey)	170
Follow-up rate (N=370)	46%
Average followup (SD) days	121 (47)
Average Age (SD) years	44 (12)
Female	42%
Chronic greater 3 years	35%
Prior surgery	14%

Hospital Surgery Indicators	
One Day Length of Stay	69%
Discharged to Home	91%
Average Charges	$7,721

Costs

Work Lost	
Missed work (28 weeks average)	54%
On leave from work at followup	6%

Financial	
Receiving Worker's Compensation	17%
Litigation: Legal action pending	6%

Satisfaction

Results of treatment(s) met expectations:	
for ability to sleep	66%
for symptom relief	61%
for ability to do activities	55%
to return to work	54%

Satisfaction:	
Satisfied with treatment(s)	85%
Would choose same treatment(s)	85%

Charges: One year episode spine specific ICD-9 codes

Spine Center		Outpatient		Inpatient	
Professional	$48,481	Diagnostic Radiology	$63,498	Surgical	$1,525,132
Physical Therapist	$71,032	Neurosurgery	$158,411	Inpatient	$2,810,156
		Orthopaedics	$160,987	Other	$737,737
		Pain Clinic	$34,769		
		Office, urgent, other	$32,918		
Total	$119,513		$450,583		$5,073,025	$5,643,121

Median per patient $13,330
Average $15,995 (SD $10,818)
Range $169 to $74,339

Figure 9-3. Clinical Value Compass data on a cohort of the Spine Center's patients with herniated disk can be used by staff to set priorities for clinical program improvement, monitoring success, fostering patient choice, shared decision making, and public transparency.

Administratively based at the University of Vermont Medical School and Fletcher-Allen Health System, the network brings together practice sites that are extremely diverse with regard to geographic location (four continents are represented), unit size, and sociodemographic mix of patients served. Some NICUs are based in major academic health centers and others in community hospitals. Despite this diversity, VON member sites share core values concerning the delivery of high-quality care, participation in educational and research activities, and collection of standardized data on very low birth weight (VLBW) infants. Sites foster shared habits of evidence-based practice, systems thinking, collaborative learning, and changing for improvement.[5]

Participating NICUs collaborate in original research and in dissemination of evidence-based best practices.[6]

Members can also participate in annual educational events and in multiyear clinical learning collaboratives, including a groundbreaking demonstration project to design "Your Ideal NICU," as described in the next section. A major VON resource is its collection of comparative clinical performance (benchmarking) data on care processes and outcomes in all member NICUs. To realize the dream of optimized clinical care, VON practitioners can use real-world data to answer this central question: "Which NICUs have the best outcomes in the world, and what are they doing to achieve these superior results?"

Outcomes measurement is thus central to VON's research/improvement mission. From the outset, the network developed standard metrics to define vital clinical outcomes—mortality and morbidity associated with premature birth. To expand the scope of this outcomes database and to

FIGURE 9-4. **A Web Page on the Quality of Care for Spine Center Patients as Publicly Reported on the Health System's Web Site**

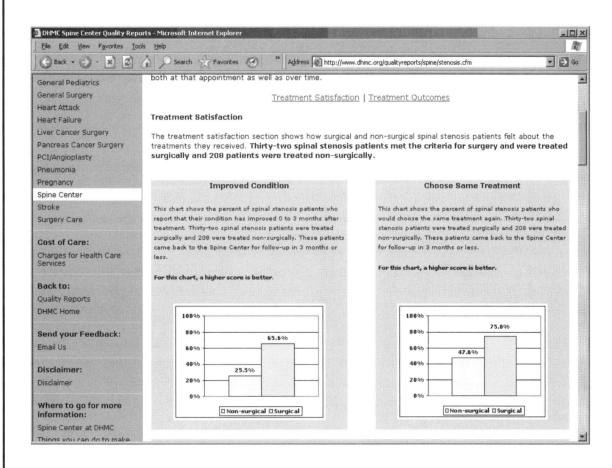

Figure 9-4. The figure depicts performance data as displayed on DHMC's publicly accessible Web site. The data are based on 61 patients with spinal stenosis who were treated surgically and 333 patients who were treated nonsurgically between January 2000 and December 2006. Source: Dartmouth-Hitchcock Medical Center: *Spinal Stenosis: Treatment Satisfaction and Outcomes.* http://www.dhmc.org/qualityreports/spine/stenosis.cfm#outcomes (accessed Jun. 27, 2007).

generate balanced measures that are relevant to families, clinical teams, institutions, and society, VON has embraced the methods and modeling of the Clinical Value Compass.

Innovation: Novel Application of Clinical Value Compass Concepts

The Clinical Value Compass, which has been used in DHMC's ICN since 1992 for infants 1,500 grams, has facilitated clarification, monitoring, and achievement of specific outcomes that matter most to premature infants and their families (Figure 9-5, page 124). In 2004, VON launched the "Your Ideal NICU" program, which was designed to dramatically improve care in NICUs at

DHMC and the 11 other health care organizations that competed for the opportunity to be part of this new program. As part of the "Your Ideal NICU" start-up activity, two of the authors [E.C.N., W.H.E.] began work with an interdisciplinary task force to design, test, and implement a Clinical Value Compass for VLBW infants. The intention was to pilot test this value compass with a subset of participating sites and then to refine it for future use by all VON members.

Methods: How It Works

The current VON VLBW Clinical Value Compass (for infants 500–1,500 grams) (Figure 9-6, page 125) presents

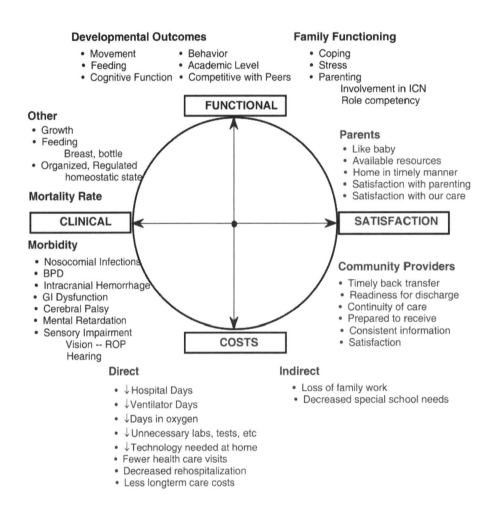

FIGURE 9-5. The Original Very Low Birth Weight (≤ 1,500 gram) Infant Clinical Value Compass Developed by the Dartmouth Intensive Care Nursery*

OUTCOMES: BABIES ≤ 1500 GRAMS

Developmental Outcomes
- Movement
- Feeding
- Cognitive Function
- Behavior
- Academic Level
- Competitive with Peers

Family Functioning
- Coping
- Stress
- Parenting
  Involvement in ICN
  Role competency

FUNCTIONAL

Other
- Growth
- Feeding
  Breast, bottle
- Organized, Regulated
  homeostatic state

Parents
- Like baby
- Available resources
- Home in timely manner
- Satisfaction with parenting
- Satisfaction with our care

Mortality Rate

CLINICAL   **SATISFACTION**

Morbidity
- Nosocomial Infections
- BPD
- Intracranial Hemorrhage
- GI Dysfunction
- Cerebral Palsy
- Mental Retardation
- Sensory Impairment
  Vision -- ROP
  Hearing

Community Providers
- Timely back transfer
- Readiness for discharge
- Continuity of care
- Prepared to receive
- Consistent information
- Satisfaction

COSTS

Direct
- ↓Hospital Days
- ↓Ventilator Days
- ↓Days in oxygen
- ↓Unnecessary labs, tests, etc
- ↓Technology needed at home
- Fewer health care visits
- Decreased rehospitalization
- Less longterm care costs

Indirect
- Loss of family work
- Decreased special school needs

Figure 9-5. The Infant Clinical Value Compass has facilitated clarification, monitoring, and achievement of specific outcomes that matter most to premature infants and their families.
* BPD, broncopulmonary dysplasia; GI, gastrointestinal; ROP, retinopathy of prematurity.

the four conventional quadrants (clinical, functional, satisfaction, and costs), as described in previous chapters of this book. Each participating NICU collects and submits data on the basis of written protocols. Data sets are sent to a central VON location for analysis and distribution. Sites receive an annual feedback report that describes local performance in absolute and relative terms, that is, in comparison to other participating NICUs. This feedback report will soon be formatted to cover the four quadrants

of the value compass framework:
- **Clinical** outcomes data for VLBW infants reflect mortality, morbidity, and treatment complications experienced during the NICU stay. Standard operational definitions are used to determine the presence or absence of clinical conditions and the values of clinical measures.
- **Functional** outcomes for premature infants are currently assessed using a special "transitions" survey

completed by parents a few weeks after discharge. This survey queries basic activities of both baby and family in the context of the potentially challenging transition to home. This short-term functional assessment will eventually be supplemented by surveys of both intermediate (age six months to two years post-discharge) and longer-term outcomes.

- **Satisfaction** assessment focuses on parental perceptions of care by NICU staff and on perceptions of their own participation in this care. Feedback is collected via an Internet-based survey (www.howsyourbaby.com) developed by William H. Edwards and John H. Wasson that was specifically designed for parents of preterm infants receiving NICU care.
- The VON Value Compass defines two cost metrics:

length of NICU stay is used as a proxy for direct medical care costs, whereas parents' evaluation of overall financial burden (including time lost from work, and so on) serves as a marker for indirect social costs. These latter data are collected in the "howsyourbaby" Internet survey.

Displays and Utility: What It Looks Like and How It's Used

For more than a decade, clinicians and staff at the DHMC ICN have used the Clinical Value Compass (Figure 9-5) to (1) clarify general goals and to specify important outcomes, (2) set priorities for improving results, and (3) communicate with patients, colleagues, and other stakeholders about achievements in high-quality, safe, cost-

---

FIGURE 9-6. The Current Vermont Oxford Network Very Low Birth Weight (500–1,500 grams) Infant Clinical Value Compass*

Value Compass 500-1500 grams

Center: Woman's Hospital   **Year: 2003**

Patient Mix (Jan-Dec)

	n	%
Patients (501-1500 grams)	173	
Birth Weight <750	37	21
Birth Weight <1000	78	45
GA < 26 weeks	36	21
	%	%-tile rank
Inborn	95	74
Male	52	56
Multiple Birth	27	52
SGA	17	29
Antenatal Steroids	72	44
Prenatal Care	98	62
Race: Black	64	93
Hispanic	1	21
White	35	24
Asian	1	39
Native American		

Functional Status

Infant: 2-3 wk after discharge	n	%	Family: 2-3 wk after discharge	n	%
Feeding			Adaptation		
Sleeping			Anxiety		
Crying			Depressed		
Ability to calm			Social		
Unscheduled care			Activities of daily living		
			Parents know baby		
			Emotional attachment		

	Infants Assessed			Functional Status (% of those Assessed)		
					Disturbance/Impairment	
	N	# eligible	%	Normal	Mild-Moderate	Moderate-Severe
Health: 18-24 mos.						
Growth						
Vision	76	159	48	78	21	1
Hearing	157	159	99	114	14	29
General Health						
Development: 18-24 mos.						
Motor	16	159	10	56	31	13
Cognitive	3	159	2	0	100	0

Clinical Outcomes

	%	%-tile rank	SMR	95%CI
Mortality	9	18	0.65	0.35-0.94
	%	%-tile rank	3-yr adj ratio	95%CI
Death or morbidity	55	56	1.09	1.02-1.16
Chronic Lung Disease	42	82	1.46	1.34-1.59
Nosocomial Sepsis	15	35	0.85	0.69-1.01
Severe IVH	9	47	1.02	0.73-1.32
Severe ROP	10	53	1	0.72-1.28
NEC	5	62	1.34	0.99-1.69
Pneumothorax	5	58	1.21	0.83-1.59

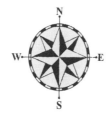

Satisfaction

Met expectations: Discharge	n	%
Parents know baby	15	47
Parents participate in care	15	80
Parents made own decisions	15	53
Satisfaction: Discharge		
Quality ="Excellent"	15	80
Parents would recommend this hospital	15	100
Parents perceived infant experienced pain	15	13
Satisfaction: 2-3 wk after discharge		
Baby prepared for discharge		
Parent ready to care for baby		
Involved in descisions regarding discharge		
How well did unit prepare for discharge		
Connection with community resources		

Costs

	n	%
Parents have financial concerns	15	13
	days	%-tile rank
Adjusted length of stay	53	27

Figure 9-6. The current Vermont Oxford Network (VON) Very Low Birth Weight (500–1,500 grams) Infant Clinical Value Compass presents data for the four quadrants—clinical, functional, satisfaction, and costs. * GA, gestational age; SGA, suspected gestational age; IVH, intraventricular hemorrhage; ROP, retinopathy of prematurity; HYB, How's Your Baby?; SMR, Standardized Mortality Ratio; NEC, Necrotizing Enterocolitis; CI, confidence interval. Reproduced with permission of Dynamic Clinical Systems, Inc. All rights reserved.

effective care. Use of value compass thinking has enabled ICN caregivers to develop specific improvement projects in all four quadrants:

- **Clinical:** minimizing infants' exposures to loud noises (which can impact biological outcomes), decreasing the rate of nosocomial infections, and lowering the incidence of chronic lung disease
- **Functional:** improving families' feelings of security and competency in postdischarge baby care
- **Satisfaction:** promoting parents' self-perception as "caregiving partners" with NICU staff and improving parent evaluations of care provided by NICU staff
- **Costs:** decreasing lengths of stay, reducing unnecessary diagnostic tests, and facilitating early discharge to infants' homes or community hospitals

Some of these initiatives have led to substantial and measurable improvements in outcomes related to nosocomial infections, noise exposure, and length of stay. As illustrated in Figure 9-7 (below), for example, the Dartmouth ICN recently logged more than 200 consecutive days without a single infant developing a nosocomial infection.

Recently, the DHMC ICN has become an active participant in VON's Your Ideal NICU program. Eight different priority improvement projects are now proceeding in parallel in this single unit, and the "best in the world" vision remains a serious goal.

Meanwhile, the larger network of VON practices has begun to document its own successes. The current VON Clinical Value Compass (Figure 9-6) permits expansion of

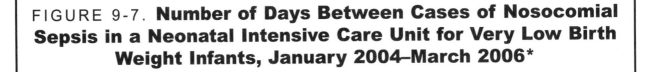

FIGURE 9-7. **Number of Days Between Cases of Nosocomial Sepsis in a Neonatal Intensive Care Unit for Very Low Birth Weight Infants, January 2004–March 2006***

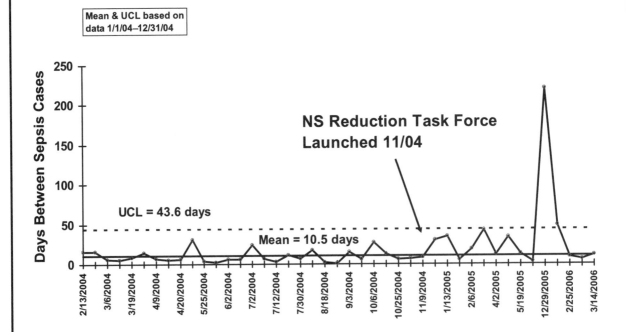

Note: The vertical axis shows the number of consecutive days that the NICU went without an infant with nosocomial sepsis.

Figure 9-7. The Dartmouth Intensive Care Nursery has logged more than 200 consecutive days without a single infant developing a nosocomial infection. * SPC, statistical process control; UCL, upper control limit; NS, nosocomial sepsis.

outcome measures available for comparative benchmarking and improvement. "Your Ideal NICU" program activities, based in part on value compass thinking, are yielding dramatic results at a number of sites. Improvements have been documented in such domains as parent-infant bonding, effective use of evidence-based protocols, coordinated handoffs for incoming and outgoing infants, and (as described previously) decreased nosocomial infections.

To introduce participating centers to new value compass methods, VON has sponsored a six-session, distance learning program facilitated by a Web communication company, and 50 NICUs have enrolled. The first session introduces the Clinical Value Compass, and the next four sessions "circle" its four points. Between sessions, participants engage in "translational homework," adapting general ideas and methods to their own clinical settings, constructing local value compasses and selecting key outcomes in each quadrant for analysis and intervention. In the final collective session, individual sites present their progress reports and discuss specific follow-up projects to sustain and to extend initial improvements.

Case 3. The Institute for Healthcare Improvement's (IHI's) Whole System Measures

Background: The Need for Innovation

In 2001, IHI, with support from the Robert Wood Johnson Foundation, launched the Pursuing Perfection Program (P3), a new initiative to create model health care delivery systems capable of achieving unprecedented levels of excellence.[7,8] Using a competitive grant application process, the program selected a small number of health systems in the United States and Europe to begin this "perfection work" in a swift, intelligent, and transparent manner.

At approximately the same time, a larger network of more than 100 health systems was being developed, again with IHI leadership and support, to test and share innovations in a collaborative manner somewhat analogous to the VON. This new learning community, called IMPACT, brought together large numbers of subscribing health systems committed to both implementation and communication of targeted improvements in health care delivery systems.[9]

The founders of both P3 and IMPACT recognized that the innovative work of transforming health care required performance metrics that were themselves innovative. Many outcome variables can be described that reflect specific domains of service in health care organiza-

tions, but how can the overall system of health care be measured? New metrics were needed to facilitate the assessment and improvement of systemwide quality.

Clinical Setting: Location of the Work

IHI faculty (including E.C.N.), together with health system leaders from selected P3 sites, worked together to develop a set of "whole system measures" (WSMs) that would inform the program's greater transformational efforts. These measures were initially developed and tested in Sweden, the United Kingdom, and the United States. Jönköping (Sweden), East Lancashire (United Kingdom), and McLeod Regional Medical Center, Geisinger Medical Center, St. Johns Mercy Health Care, and Thedacare (United States) constituted the initial test sites.

Innovation: Definitions of Quality

A member WSM task force was assembled to develop, test, and implement a small set of measures that summarized, in a balanced manner, the quality of care delivered by entire health care systems. The Institute of Medicine's (IOM's) then-recently published *Quality Chasm* report identified six broad dimensions of care deemed essential for achievement of overall quality—high-quality must be safe, timely, effective, efficient, equitable, and patient-centered.[10] The WSM task force built these six dimensions into its own operational definitions of systemwide health care quality. After considering several potential WSM metrics, it ultimately selected a smaller set most appropriate for pilot testing in large and diverse health systems. Prototype measures were defined and data collection and display methods were refined, so that use of WSMs would be practicable and meaningful at all P3 and IMPACT sites.

Methods: How It Works

The six test sites conducted a pilot test of 10 potential quality measures in 2003 and 2004. On the basis of initial experience with these proposed measures (including their utility in data collection, analysis, reporting, and stimulation of specific improvement work), Version 1.0 of the WSM Tool Kit was produced. This kit incorporated nine measures that cut across the six IOM quality categories and included both inpatient and outpatient domains of clinical service.

Subsequently, in late 2004 and early 2005, a larger group of 30 health systems collected data and measured their progress using these same WSMs. Lessons learned from their work, and progress in the field of health care quality improvement prompted the task force to revise its initial metrics.[11] Version 2.0 of the WSM tool kit includes the following 10 measures (and specifies their means of collection):

1. **Safe:** Adverse Events: Inpatient and Outpatient (local record review data)
2. **Safe:** Work Days Lost (local Occupational Safety and Health Administration report data)
3. **Effective:** Hospital Standardized Mortality Ratio (national discharge data set)
4. **Effective:** Unadjusted Raw Mortality (local record review)
5. **Effective:** Functional Outcomes (local patient survey)
6. **Effective:** 30-Day Readmission Percentage (local record review)
7. **Patient-Centered:** Patient Satisfaction—Inpatient and Outpatient (local patient survey)
8. **Timely:** Third-Next Available Appointment—Primary Care and Specialty Care (local record review)
9. **Efficient:** Inpatient Days During the Last Six Months of Life (national discharge data set)
10. **Efficient:** Health Care Costs per Capita for a Region (national discharge data set)

The sixth IOM quality dimension, equity, is not monitored in a single metric. Instead, this variable is assessed via stratification of the other measures, when possible, into relevant subpopulations. Thus, available data permit stratification by gender, age, or racial grouping. This capacity permits meaningful assessment of equity, in terms of service delivery and outcome distribution, within and across health care systems.

The task force attempted to balance scope and rigor with practical field conditions and logistical issues. Participating health systems are responsible for collection of 7 of the 10 identified measures, and national data sets provide information for the other three. Standard protocols guide collection and calculation of all values.

Local data are submitted to IHI by individual health systems, and national data are sent by health services research organizations. IHI creates a master database for use in monitoring and comparative benchmarking. These data are formatted to illustrate point-in-time values and demonstrate trends over time.

Displays and Utility: What It Looks Like and How It's Used

The task force, which experimented with several methods of data display, found the value compass approach to be especially useful for development of a "dashboard" to monitor systemwide performance. Figure 9-8 (page 129) illustrates a typical value compass–based array of "dashboard" or "instrument panel" data, adapted for use with WSM metrics. The layout of this dashboard reflects value compass thinking by visually connecting process drivers with a balanced set of health outcomes. Site-specific data from the Geisinger Health System are presented in Figure 9-9 (page 130). A cardinal virtue of value compass display is its capacity to communicate to users the big picture of system performance. Multiple dimensions of quality are highlighted simultaneously, so that attention to one component of care does not undermine attention to the others. Indeed, the dashboard view reminds users that creative work in one domain almost always connects to and stimulates improvement in others, and "downstream" outcomes are produced by "upstream" processes that aim to meet patients' needs.

Reflections on Advanced Applications of Practice-Based Learning and Improvement

What can we learn from these case studies? What common themes are relevant to clinicians in their own daily work of patient care, practice improvement, and professional development? Though our examples progress from local to regional to, in the case of the IHI Whole System Measures, global application of improvement methods and principles, we recognize here the same tools and concepts that have been explored throughout the current volume. Several points warrant specific consideration:

- **Innovative Approaches to Data Collection Must Be Built into Daily Care Processes.** Proper measurement of clinical outcomes requires not only technical expertise but also tireless ingenuity. Successful implementation of Spine Center initiatives required capturing new data streams, in real time, from both patients and clinicians, and this work was facilitated by Clinical Value Compass–based "feed forward" innovations. In the VON collaborative and P3 and IMPACT networks, novel data collection and display strategies had to be designed, tested, and (importantly) coordinated with mainstream data gathering activities already in place at the mother institutions. Because such collaborations will become increasingly normative in the work of health care improvement, new information networks must seamlessly integrate complex data across multiple institutions in a user-friendly and system-compatible manner.

FIGURE 9-8. **Whole System Measures (WSM) Dashboard***

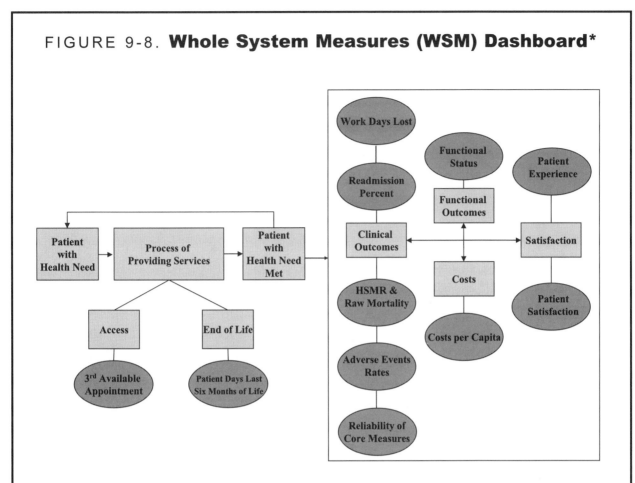

Figure 9-8. A typical value compass–based array of "dashboard" or "instrument panel" data, adapted for use with WSM metrics, is shown. The dashboard's layout reflects value compass thinking by visually connecting process drivers with a balanced set of health outcomes. * HSMR, hospital standardized mortality ratio. Source: Institute for Healthcare Improvement. Used with permission.

- **Consideration of Outcomes Must Be Balanced and Inclusive.** The VON NICU case reminds us, especially, that illness and health are not defined simply in terms of the target patient's biological parameters but that they extend to functional, psychological, and economic experiences of all participants, including parents and community caregivers. Clinicians at the Spine Center understand that chronic back pain affects all facets of life, and leaders of the P3 project acknowledge multiple dimensions of care in their systemwide assessment. Again, the Clinical Value Compass builds such multidimensionality into both daily care and longer-term strategic planning.

- **Increased Transparency Is a Fact of Life to Be Embraced (Rather than Resisted) in the Evolving Health Care System.** As discussed in Chapter 1, evidence-based metrics are increasingly monitored by employers, regulators, payers, and the public, and this trend will certainly continue in the foreseeable future.[12–14] Transparency can be turned to collective advantage by individual clinicians and entire health systems in the work of health care improvement. Thus, at Dartmouth's Spine Center, public access to performance data promotes informed decision making by patients and families. At VON, collective data sharing permits comparative benchmarking to achieve better outcomes across participating sites. In the IHI's P3 practices, similar reporting of systemwide outcomes permits dissemination of best strategies for care.

- **Practice-Based Learning is Built Into the Work of Improvement Itself.** Adult learners in general, and maturing practitioners in particular, learn best (and learn continuously) through an active and iterative

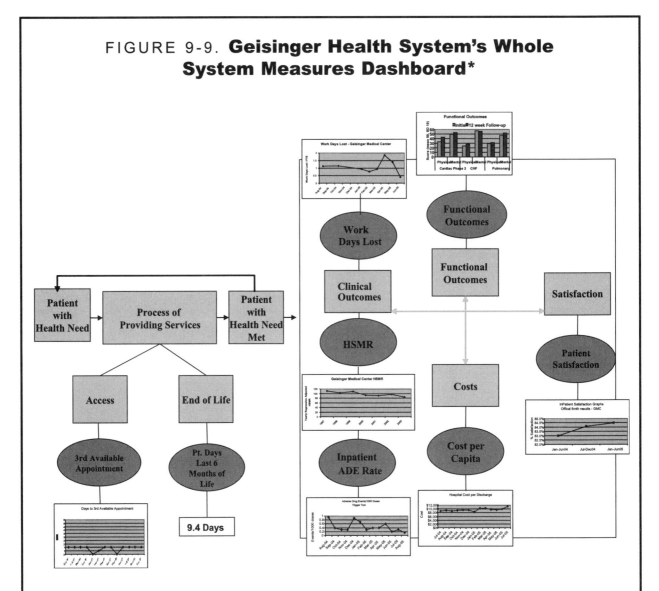

FIGURE 9-9. **Geisinger Health System's Whole System Measures Dashboard***

Figure 9-9. Geisinger Health System's Whole System Measures Dashboard communicates the big picture of system performance. *HSMR, hospital standardized mortality ratio; ADE, adverse drug event.

process that includes self-generation of ideas, thoughtful implementation of test interventions, careful assessment (including quantitative measurement) of specific consequences, and regular reflection on the process itself. These are indeed the same activities that support clinical improvement work at both microsystem and macrosystem levels. Through processes of increasingly refined trial and error, or trial and success, dedicated practitioners at the Spine Center, the VON collaborative, and the IHI's P3 and IMPACT networks, are learning in the field how to improve spine care, how to raise the bar for NICU performance, and how to measure and support systemwide clinical improvement.

- As we asserted in Chapter 1, health care improvement is indeed the work of everyone. But we now see that this "everyone" includes not only "each individual" striving for professional excellence but also the collective "everyone," working together in expanding levels of collaboration. The Spine Center and Dartmouth ICN excel not only because they are staffed by talented and committed individuals but also because these individuals bring varied perspectives, skills, and experiences to the common tasks of patient care and system improvement. At the VON collaborative and the P3 and IMPACT, best ideas are shared to the mutual advantage of all participating practices; "it is exponentially easier to improve together than it is alone."[9]

Final Reflections: The Work of Everyone

We thus come full circle to the message with which this book began. As depicted in Figure 1-2 (page 5), practice-based learning and improvement is the work of everyone, which is to say, the work of each of us individually and all of us collectively. We strive together to achieve the common and mutually supportive goals of better patient outcomes, better system performance, and better professional development. The Clinical Value Compass clarifies and coordinates the wide range of outcomes available for improvement work, and the knowledge and skills rehearsed throughout this book (and described in the Clinical Improvement Equation, Chapter 1) empower practitioners to optimize both microsystem and macrosystem performance, even as they support practice-based learning and professional development.[14]

There is enough work to be done, and enough variety of work, to meet the various talents, interests, and personal inclinations of all heath care professionals. As we have emphasized repeatedly, improvement work can be practiced independently or collectively, and in small informal learning groups or large multidisciplinary collaborations. As we demonstrate in the present chapter, this same work can be targeted to settings that are local or regional or even international. Some of us will pursue our improvement mission in the context of solo practice, building simple but meaningful changes into personal work routines. Others will direct attention to spine centers or NICUs, hospitals or regional networks, or entire health care systems.

Some of us (including authors and editors of this book) will endeavor to develop the educational infrastructure required to advance health professionals' competence in practice-based learning and improvement. We must also commit ourselves to the iterative work of testing, assessment, and reflection, as principles of and experiences in practice-based learning and improvement are introduced early and reinforced throughout the medical school curriculum and residency education programs.

In this spirit, we invite readers of *Practice-Based Learning and Improvement: A Clinical Improvement Action Guide*, Second Edition, to guide us in our own continual learning. Our hope is that practitioners will experiment with methods we have described and will communicate with us regarding successes and failures, adaptations, and further innovations. Correspondence can be addressed to Eugene C. Nelson, D.Sc., eugene.c.nelson@hitchcock.org, Dartmouth-Hitchcock Medical Center, 1 Medical Center Drive, Lebanon, NH 03756.

As in any cycle of continuous learning and improvement, we may ask again here, at the end of this book, "Where (*again*) do we begin…?" The poet David Whyte reminds us, "Start close in… Start with the ground [we] know, the pale ground beneath [our] feet." With each new observation made, each improvement tested, refined, and tested again, this ground becomes more comfortable and familiar, and at the same time more inviting to continuous exploration.

References

1. Whyte D.: *River Flow: New & Selected Poems 1984–2007*. Langley, WA: Many Rivers Press, 2007.
2. Weinstein J., et al.: Designing an ambulatory clinical practice for outcomes improvement: From vision to reality—the Spine Center at Dartmouth-Hitchcock, year one. *Qual Manag Health Care* 8:1–20, Winter 2000.
3. Ware J.E. Jr.: *SF-36® Health Survey Update*. http://www.sf-36.org/tools/sf36.shtml (accessed Jun. 1, 2007).
4. Weinstein J., et al.: Surgical vs. nonoperative treatment for lumbar disk herniation: The Spine Patient Outcomes Research Trial (SPORT) observational cohort. *JAMA* 296:2451–2459, Nov. 22, 2006.
5. Vermont Oxford Network: *About Vermont Oxford Network*. http://www.vtoxford.org/home.aspx?p=about/index.htm (last accessed Jan. 31, 2007).
6. Edwards W., et al.: The effect of prophylactic ointment therapy on nosocomial sepsis rates and skin integrity in infants with birth weights of 501 to 1000 g. *Pediatrics* 113:1195–1203, May 2004.
7. Nolan T.W., et al.: Large-scale system change improves outcomes: The Pursuing Perfection program. *Journal of Clinical Outcomes Management* 12:569–576, Nov. 2005.
8. Institute for Healthcare Improvement: *IMPACT: Improvement/Action*. http://www.ihi.org/IHI/Programs/IMPACTNetwork/ (accessed Jun. 4, 2007).
9. Institute of Medicine: *Crossing the Quality Chasm: A New Health System for the 21st Century*. Washington, DC: National Academy Press, 2001.
10. Lloyd R., Martin L., Nelson E.: *IHI's Whole System Measures Tool Kit: Version 2.0*. Institute for Healthcare Improvement (IHI), Jul. 18, 2006. http://www.ihi.org/NR/rdonlyres/0848B270-EA39-4B90-9AC2-2C8DF3A1379D/3644/IHIWholeSystemMeasuresToolkitV271906.pdf (accessed Jun. 4, 2007).
11. Institute of Medicine: *Performance Measurement: Accelerating Improvement*. Washington, DC: National Academy Press, 2001.
12. National Quality Forum (NQF): *National Priorities for Healthcare Quality Measurement and Reporting*. Washington, DC: NQF, 2004.
13. National Quality Forum (NQF): *National Voluntary Consensus Standards for Hospital Care: An Initial Performance Measurement Set*. Washington, DC: NQF, 2003.
14. Batalden P.B., Godfrey M.M., Nelson E.C.: *Quality by Design: A Clinical Microsystems Approach*. San Francisco: Jossey-Bass, 2007.

Afterword

David Leach

What one book would you like to have with you if you were stranded on a desert island? G.K. Chesterton's answer: "Thomas's Guide to Practical Shipbuilding." [1]

This book, developed by Eugene Nelson, Paul Batalden, and Joel Lazar, is an important one. Unlike most practical guides, *Practice-Based Learning and Improvement: A Clinical Improvement Action Guide,* Second Edition, reads easily, is based on real examples, and could actually help us get off the island on which we currently seem to be stuck. The authors have been deeply engaged in the work of improving patient care, in some cases for decades, and speak with an authenticity that is both clear and rare.

In reflecting on the book, I found myself reflecting on my own experience with improvement work. Several years ago Paul Batalden suggested that I improve something. At the time I was a busy practitioner in a large health care system, and I decided to attempt to return all phone calls within one day. He told me to gather some data, taught me how to make a simple run chart, clarified common and special cause variation, and taught me how to draw a Pareto chart and a fishbone diagram. Informed by the data, I actually improved. Then I decided to improve patient care.

I met Gene Nelson; he asked me my aim. I told him that I wanted to improve patient care. He taught me how useless, if noble, such an aim was, and then asked a set of clarifying questions that got me from "improve patient care" to "improve the care of diabetic patients" to "improve the care of my diabetic patients" to "increase the number of diabetic patients in my practice with a glycolated hemoglobin of 8.0% or less." At that time I did not know the data about my diabetic patients as a group—I only saw them one by one in the clinic.

Paul and Gene then taught me about the Clinical Value Compass. If all of my diabetic patients had a normal glycolated hemoglobin but had numerous hypoglycemic reactions or were unable to work, or were miserable, or were broke because of unmanageable medical expenses, I had not improved care. This, of course, makes a great deal of sense, but the simplicity and clarity of the Clinical Value Compass invited a balanced set of measures that made it possible to determine if a change was actually an improvement.

I learned that improvement begins with "I" and that the first step was the hardest—changing myself. Things that helped included being clear about the aim and measuring and displaying a balanced set of data. I also learned that change and improvement involve talking with others. Then it got really interesting.

Describing the various sets of relationships involved in patient care as micro-, meso-, and macrosystems identifies the relevant conversational units and creates a sense of belonging that is the foundation for accountability. For me, inquiring into the observations of the various participants in the microsystem (or meso- or macrosystems) was a good way to begin. That was true in clinical practice and when I was a residency program director, a designated institutional official, and finally at the Accreditation Council for Graduate Medical Education. Conversations designed to create a common vision were helpful, but more interesting—and more difficult—were the conversations designed to clarify the current reality. People differed. Eliciting diverse views of the current reality was made easier by drawing process maps—the more detailed the better. It helped to have all process owners present. It was tedious but essential and documented a larger and more inclusive view of the current reality than any one participant could provide.

It is said that people resist change, but my own experience has been that people are attracted to change. People want to understand the truth, to help patients, and most of all to do something creative and even beautiful. The key to unlocking those native tendencies is to host conversations that are both hospitable and charged. Nominal group and rank ordering techniques, DeBono's thinking-hat exercises, appreciative inquiry, and other techniques were helpful supplements to discussion. They disrupted the usual hierarchical communication patterns and made it easy for everyone to participate.

The power of transparency of the processes and the results of improvement efforts cannot be overstated. It lets all involved use a common reference point and begins to spread the news to others. Of the many things in health care that need to be improved, few are as core as trust. Hospital Web sites hosting obviously exaggerated claims might change perceptions, but they do not change reality and they diminish patient trust. However, Web sites that display accurate and comparative clinical outcome data encourage both improvement and trust.

Two of the several useful concepts and tools in this book are the use of the Clinical Value Compass to guide and judge improvement in health professional development and the simple but very powerful statement that the quality of patient care, the quality of health professional formation, and the quality of system performance are inextricably linked. Good health professional formation cannot occur in the absence of good patient care, and neither can occur in systems not designed to enable and facilitate both. Yet how many faculty can actually document their own patient care outcomes? How many academic medical centers display accurate and comparative patient care outcome data on their public Web site? The data are not encouraging. It has been reported that health care known to be good is only delivered about 54% of the time—and only 2%–3% if interventions are bundled.[2] No one knows the comparable numbers for health professional formation or for system performance—but everyone has a story to tell about how much improvement is needed.

The task of improving patient care and health professional formation is helped by organizing the work around the five knowledge domains detailed in the book—generalizable knowledge, context-specific knowledge, integrative knowledge (adapting for best fit), executing change, and creating balanced sets of measures. The knowledge domains construct is extremely useful; it can be applied to the care for an individual patient, to the formation of a resident-learner, and to the improvement of graduate medical education at the national level.

Although not explicit in the book, one could construct "the seven habits of effective improvers": (1) recognize that health care is everybody's business—don't work in isolation; (2) begin with the end in mind—get the aim right; (3) clarify the current reality with all who work in the system being improved; (4) use the Clinical Value Compass to organize measurements; (5) use this *Clinical Improvement Action Guide*; (6) host clarifying conversations using well-established tools for managing small groups; (7) work with rather than against nature—remove barriers to the natural tendencies to discern and tell the truth to help patients and residents and to do something creative and even beautiful.

The eighth habit should be to enjoy the work; it is noble work. This book provides tools; it is time to apply those tools in various contexts—to move from novice to competent and to expert and master. The world needs your help.

References

1. The Blog of the American Chesterton Society: Aug. 11, 2006. http://americanchestertonsociety.blogspot.com/2006/08/i-gkc-posting-today-was-tagged-for.html (accessed Jun. 5, 2007).
2. Schuster M.A., McGlynn E.A., Brook R.H.: How good is the quality of health care in the United States? *Milbank Q* 83(4):843–895, 2005.

IMPROVING CARE: CLINICAL IMPROVEMENT WORKSHEETS

Eugene C. Nelson

Leading an Improvement Study Group: Planning and Conducting a Meeting

Description of an Improvement Study Group

An Improvement Study Group is a group of individuals who come together to share their learning about improvement in specific work settings. The groups form by mutual attraction—individuals perceive a safe setting in which they can freely explore new ideas and through which they can both give and receive support. Participants generally use a common framework as they design and test changes, and all members can choose to focus on the same general area of improvement (for example, access, obesity, diabetes mellitus), although each person implements his or her own change project.

Ground Rules for Getting Started

Participants can agree on rules to facilitate the group process. Here is starter set of such rules:

- Help each other learn.
- Reflect together on the work of improving care…start with what seems to work.
- Use questions to clarify—not to guide.
- Keep the space open for inquiry.
- Use conflicting viewpoints to understand better.
- Keep exploring questions that are most difficult to answer.
- Have some fun.

General Guidance

- Expect that people will come and go during the life of the study group.
- Make sure that everyone knows one another.
- Keep the group to fewer than 10 persons, and keep meetings to no more than one hour in length. Make the meetings easy to attend.
- Consider ending the group periodically.
- Meet frequently enough to prevent the need for exhausting re-caps at the start of each session.

Typical Meeting Structure

1. Share general aim and meeting process.
2. Share general model for testing a change (for example, Clinical Improvement Worksheet for Individuals).
3. Present a focused case study—keep this rotating, so everyone has a chance to present.
   a. Walk through the worksheet as far as members have gotten; share the data.
   b. Ask questions—what still needs to be learned in the specific improvement project? Use prompting questions to assist in reflection. Try for open, honest inquiry. Resist questions that hide advice within them.
   c. Reflect on lessons learned (by presenter and by others in the group).
   d. Recap the lessons learned.
4. Recap questions—itemized on a flip chart.
5. Plan for the next meeting.
6. Feedback: What went well during meeting, and what could be improved? (Note: feedback and agenda plan for next meeting could go on a single sheet of paper, which can be posted by the leader/facilitator of the next meeting, eliminating the need for an additional transcriber.)

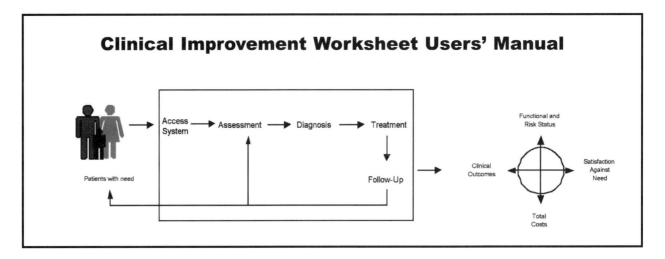

Clinical Improvement Worksheet Users' Manual

Introduction

This manual for the Clinical Improvement Worksheet is intended to be used by individual clinicians for practice-based learning and improvement (*see* Clinical Improvement Worksheet for Individuals [Figure A-1, page 137; Figure A-2, page 138]) or by clinical groups who aim to improve care—such as members of a neonatal intensive care unit (NICU), a family practice center or an obstetrics (OB) practice (*see* Clinical Improvement Worksheet for Teams [Figure A-3, page 139; Figure A-4, page 140; Figure A-5, page 141; and Figure A-6, page 142).

This worksheet can also be used by special, interdisciplinary task forces that strive to increase quality and to reduce costs during episodes of care that extend across different microsystems. For example, a patient with heart failure might receive care from outpatient, inpatient, and home health microsystems over time; the need exists to optimize care both within and between these semi-independent clinical microsystems.

Instructions

The following paragraphs offer brief instructions and comments for each part of the Clinical Improvement Worksheet. To clarify instructions, the steps of Side A are numbered 1 through 6, and the steps of Side B are lettered A through H. Although the instructions and comments are provided in a typical linear sequence, it is not necessary to strictly follow this order of steps. The Clinical Improvement Worksheet for Individuals is shorter and simpler than the Worksheet for Teams. Therefore, users of the Clinical Improvement Worksheet for Individuals can skip over the steps in this Manual that are not included in the version for solo improvement work.

Getting Started

The top section of Side B has space for recording who participate in the improvement activity. Group members might wish to designate roles such as leader, facilitator, coach, administrative support, data specialist, and senior leadership champion.

Team Members (Who Should Work on This Improvement?)

Consider these guidelines when determining who to engage in the improvement work:

a. Limit the number of members to eight or fewer people for positive group dynamics.

b. Select frontline people who are familiar with key elements of the core process.

c. Reflect diverse areas of expertise and knowledge by including interdisciplinary staff as well as patients and family.

d. Designate a leader who is credible and responsible for the clinical process.

e. If the group is new to improvement work, consider using an experienced improvement coach or advisor if this expertise is available.

Tips: Select a set time and day of the week to meet on a regular basis to plan and oversee the first improvement cycle. Structured meeting agendas are recommended.[1] The participants can be a naturally occurring work group (people who normally work together such as neonatal intensive care unit staff, a family practice patient "pod," or an obstetrics practice staff) or a special ad hoc task force specifically assembled—or chartered—to work on a particular clinical topic (such as prevention of surgical

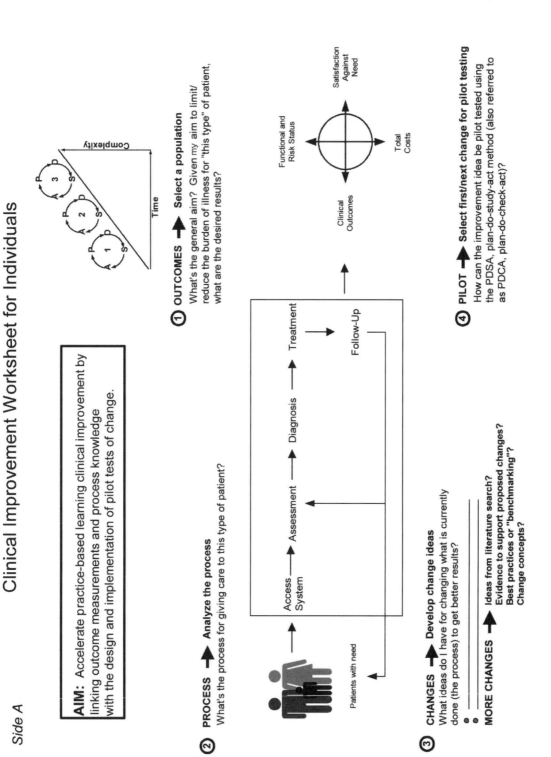

FIGURE A-1. **Clinical Improvement Worksheet for Individuals, Side A**

Side A

Clinical Improvement Worksheet for Individuals

AIM: Accelerate practice-based learning clinical improvement by linking outcome measurements and process knowledge with the design and implementation of pilot tests of change.

① OUTCOMES ➤ **Select a population**
What's the general aim? Given my aim to limit/reduce the burden of illness for "this type" of patient, what are the desired results?

② PROCESS ➤ **Analyze the process**
What's the process for giving care to this type of patient?

Access System → Assessment → Diagnosis → Treatment → Follow-Up

Patients with need

③ CHANGES ➤ **Develop change ideas**
What ideas do I have for changing what is currently done (the process) to get better results?

MORE CHANGES ➤ Ideas from literature search?
Evidence to support proposed changes?
Best practices or "benchmarking"?
Change concepts?

④ PILOT ➤ **Select first/next change for pilot testing**
How can the improvement idea be pilot tested using the PDSA, plan-do-study-act method (also referred to as PDCA, plan-do-check-act)?

Satisfaction Against Need
Functional and Risk Status
Clinical Outcomes
Total Costs

Complexity
Time

FIGURE A-2. **Clinical Improvement Worksheet for Individuals, Side B**

Side B   Clinical Improvement Worksheet for Individuals
Making a test of change

A. SELECTED CHANGE How would I describe the change that you have selected for testing?

Anyone else that _____
needs to work on _____
this with me? _____

B. AIM What is the accomplishment I seek to test? (in more specific terms?)

C. MEASURES How will I know that a change is an improvement?

D. Plan How shall the idea be tested (what, where, when, how)? What will need to be measured? Any baseline data available, needed?

E. Do What is happening/what was learned as the planned test of change was tried?

F. Study After gathering the data, analyzing it and assessing the general experience of trying out the change, what emerges? Did the original outcomes improve as planned?

G. Act What should be done to hold the gains over time, or to discontinue the test of change? What was learned?

wound infections, adolescent asthma, total joint replacement, or care of people with complex chronic problems). The participant list should not be finalized until there is a good sense of the patient population that will be targeted for improvement. In practice, it is usually necessary to make a preliminary determination of the selected population and the broad aim (see Step 1) before selecting the participants.

Side A: Ready...Aim
1. Outcomes → Select a population
To select a patient population, identify several criteria to

narrow the focus. Potential criteria include procedures or diagnoses which have high volumes, high rates of harm, high costs (including long lengths of stay), high improvement potential per case, intense market competition, high probability of achieving change, importance to stakeholders, and clinician interest.

Tips: To start the process, consider a target area in which there is both a business need and strong clinician interest. Investment of improvement work in one topic might mean foregoing work on another topic. Reviewing strategy, mission, and data on current performance versus

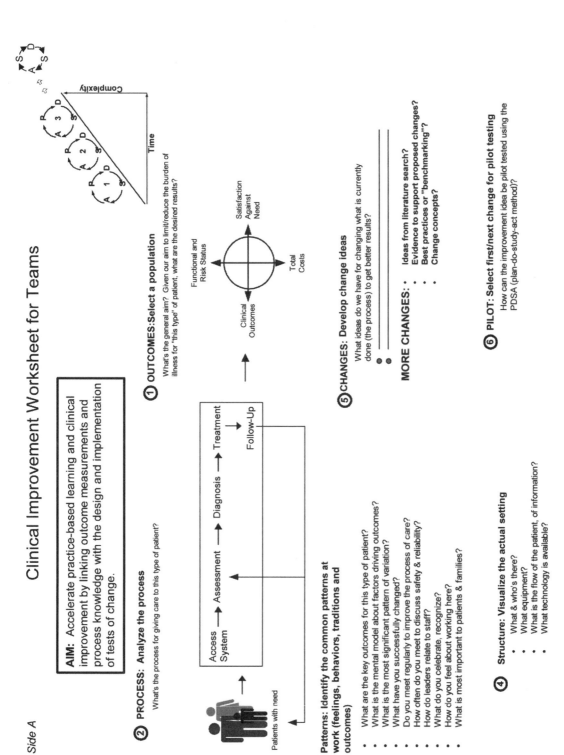

FIGURE A-3. **Clinical Improvement Worksheet for Teams, Side A**

Side A

Clinical Improvement Worksheet for Teams

AIM: Accelerate practice-based learning and clinical improvement by linking outcome measurements and process knowledge with the design and implementation of tests of change.

① **OUTCOMES: Select a population**

What's the general aim? Given our aim to limit/reduce the burden of illness for "this type" of patient, what are the desired results?

- Functional and Risk Status
- Satisfaction Against Need
- Clinical Outcomes
- Total Costs

② **PROCESS: Analyze the process**

What's the process for giving care to this type of patient?

Access System → Assessment → Diagnosis → Treatment → Follow-Up

Patients with need

③ **Patterns: Identify the common patterns at work (feelings, behaviors, traditions and outcomes)**

- What are the key outcomes for this type of patient?
- What is the mental model about factors driving outcomes?
- What is the most significant pattern of variation?
- What have you successfully changed?
- Do you meet regularly to improve the process of care?
- How often do you meet to discuss safety & reliability?
- How do leaders relate to staff?
- What do you celebrate, recognize?
- How do you feel about working here?
- What is most important to patients & families?

④ **Structure: Visualize the actual setting**

- What & who's there?
- What equipment?
- What is the flow of the patient, of information?
- What technology is available?

⑤ **CHANGES: Develop change ideas**

What ideas do we have for changing what is currently done (the process) to get better results?

MORE CHANGES:

- Ideas from literature search?
- Evidence to support proposed changes?
- Best practices or "benchmarking"?
- Change concepts?

⑥ **PILOT: Select first/next change for pilot testing**

How can the first/next change be pilot tested using the PDSA (plan-do-study-act method)?

Complexity / Time

FIGURE A-4. **Clinical Improvement Worksheet for Teams, Side B**

Side B

Clinical Improvement Worksheet for Teams
Making a test of change

A. SELECTED CHANGE How would you describe the change that you have selected for testing?

PARTICIPANTS : Who should work on this improvement?
Can patients & families be included?

1. _____ 5. _____
2. _____ 6. _____
3. _____ 7. _____
4. _____ 8. _____

RELEVANT ASPECTS OF :
- Structure
- Process
- Pattern

B. AIM What is the accomplishment we seek to test?
(in more specific terms?)

C. MEASURES How will we know that a change is an improvement?

D. Plan How shall the idea be tested (what, where, when, how)? What will need to be measured? Any baseline data available, needed? What tools and training are needed?

E. Do What is happening/what was learned as the planned test of change was tried? (structure, process, pattern)

F. Study After gathering the data, analyzing it and assessing the general experience of trying out the change, what emerges? Did the original outcomes improve as planned? Relation to structure, process, pattern?

G. Act What should be done (to structure, process, patterns) to hold the gains over time, or to discontinue the test of change? What was learned?

H. SDSA (STANDARDIZE-DO-STUDY-ACT): How do we ensure that the desired changes are standardized and practiced? What needs to be measured and monitored over time? Who will do it?

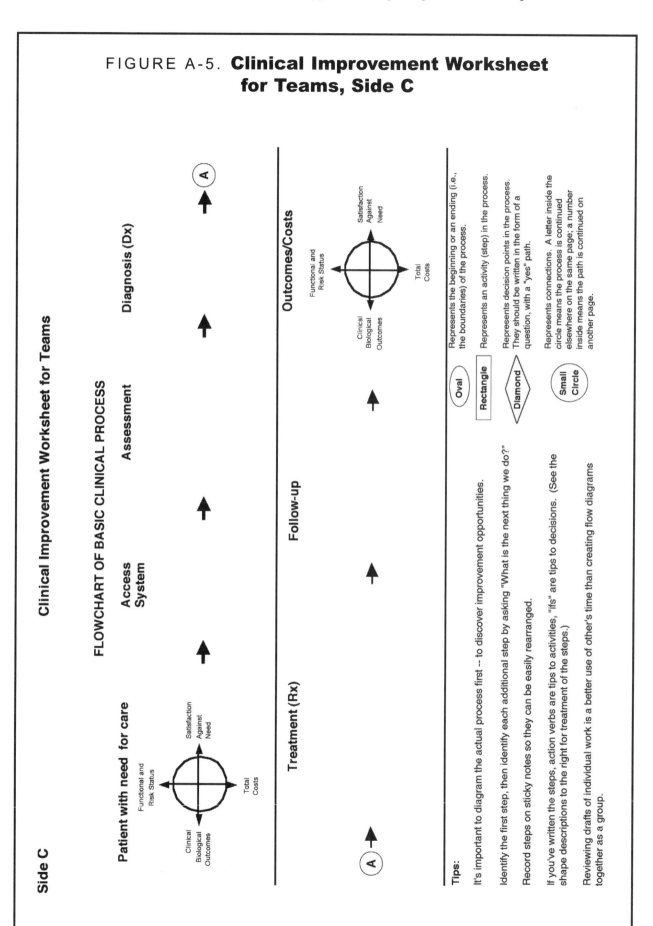

FIGURE A-5. **Clinical Improvement Worksheet for Teams, Side C**

Side C

Clinical Improvement Worksheet for Teams

FLOWCHART OF BASIC CLINICAL PROCESS

Access System · Assessment · Diagnosis (Dx)

Patient with need for care

- Functional and Risk Status
- Satisfaction Against Need
- Total Costs
- Clinical Biological Outcomes

Treatment (Rx) · Follow-up · Outcomes/Costs

- Functional and Risk Status
- Satisfaction Against Need
- Total Costs
- Clinical Biological Outcomes

(A)

Oval — Represents the beginning or an ending (i.e., the boundaries) of the process.

Rectangle — Represents an activity (step) in the process.

Diamond — Represents decision points in the process. They should be written in the form of a question, with a "yes" path.

Small Circle — Represents connections. A letter inside the circle means the process is continued elsewhere on the same page; a number inside means the path is continued on another page.

Tips:

It's important to diagram the actual process first -- to discover improvement opportunities.

Identify the first step, then identify each additional step by asking "What is the next thing we do?"

Record steps on sticky notes so they can be easily rearranged.

If you've written the steps, action verbs are tips to activities, "ifs" are tips to decisions. (See the shape descriptions to the right for treatment of the steps.)

Reviewing drafts of individual work is a better use of other's time than creating flow diagrams together as a group.

FIGURE A-6. **Clinical Improvement Worksheet for Teams, Side D**

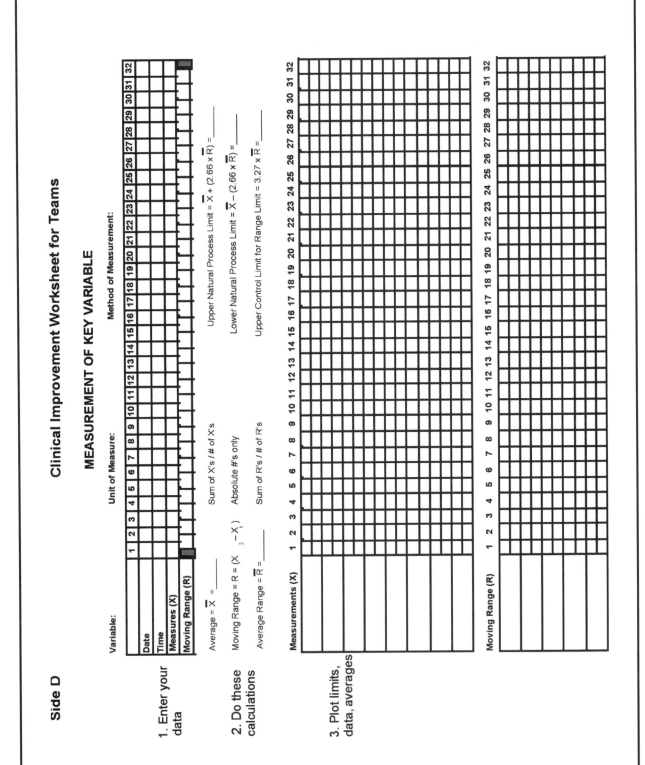

best known performance can help to identify populations for improvement work.

What's the general aim? Start with a broad statement concerning the general, long-term aim for the selected patient population. The aim statement might touch on multiple aspects of quality, safety, and costs. This aim statement can be sharpened and made more specific when preparing for the pilot tests of change.

Tips: The aim statement can indicate the name of the process, where the process starts and finishes, and what some of the expected benefits of improvement will be.

Given our aim to limit or to reduce the burden of illness for this type of patient, what are the desired results? Based on the general aim statement, brainstorm to identify potentially important clinical, functional and risk status, satisfaction, and cost outcomes for the selected patient population. Start with clinical outcomes on the Clinical Value Compass (west) and proceed to functional and risk status (north), satisfaction against need (east), and finish with total costs (south). After clarifying the meaning of each brainstormed suggestion, use multivoting to identify the one to three most important results in each area.

Tips: See Chapter 4 on measuring outcomes and costs for more detailed instructions on this step. Make a wall-sized illustration of the Clinical Value Compass (use flip-chart paper), and place the brainstormed ideas and highest-priority results onto the wall directly beside each pertinent compass point. This will build a clear, graphic model for all the team to review and refine.

2. Process → Analyze the Process

What's the process for giving care to this type of patient? Construct a flowchart of the care delivery process. Begin by specifying the process boundaries, that is, where the process should start and finish for the selected patient population. For example, the process starts when patients do "x" (for example, enter the emergency department) and the process ends when patients do "y" (for example, exit the emergency department). The participants should construct a first-draft flowchart (graphic mapping) of the delivery process. It is often wise to begin with a simple high-level flowchart (5 to 20 steps) and refine the flowchart over time. Use basic conventions of

flowcharting—ovals at the beginning and end of the process, rectangles for main action steps, diamonds for important decision points, and so on.

A patient's characteristics will tend to influence what is done for the patient as well as affect the results of care. Therefore, it is helpful to specify the patient characteristics that are most likely to have a direct impact on either what's done for the patient—in terms of clinical processes that match care with patient characteristics—or what happens to the patient in terms of outcomes. Common patient descriptors that tend to influence process or outcomes are demographics (age, gender, education), health factors (diagnosis, severity of primary diagnosis, comorbidities), and other issues such as patient's lifestyle, values, and treatment expectations.

Tips: Make the flowchart big enough for all to view it and include space for comments. Consider posting it in a place for participants and other staff members to review between meetings. Ask each participant to discuss the improvement work in general and the flowchart specifically with one or two colleagues or patients/family members (who are not participating in this particular improvement) to refine the flowchart and gain better understanding of improvement work rationale and methods. Also make a wall-sized illustration (using flip-chart pages) of the graphic elements of Side A of the worksheet showing the basic flow of the process to cover the sequence listed below:

3. Patterns → Identify the Common Patterns at Work

Common patterns at work include feelings, behaviors, traditions, norms, values, tools, techniques, outcomes, and so on. Improvement always happens in specific places. These places have special and unique cultural contexts that can be understood by examining important patterns that recur in that place. In addition, these places have particular improvement histories that reflect past attempts to make changes or to do things differently.

Tips: Discuss cultural patterns relevant to making (and sustaining!) improvements by discussing the questions on Side A listed under the "Patterns" heading. Hold a dialogue on these and related questions. This will help participants gain a shared understanding of the unique and important features of the specific contexts that they intend to learn about and make durable improvements that are built to last.

4. Structure → Visualize the Actual Setting

What and who's there? What equipment? What technology is available? Visualize what is happening "on the ground" in the specific places where the process unfolds and outcomes are made. Gain an accurate understanding of the physical and structural elements that "front-end load" the work.

> **Tips:** Use direct observation and/or participant observation methods to document important structural features of the actual settings in which the care processes are embedded, (see Appendix B for methods). What are the physical and intellectual inputs? How are space and technology used? Are there simple changes that could be made to do the following:
> • Streamline the physical layout.
> • Clean up messes or untidy places.
> • Improve the safety of the space.
> • Have needed equipment in the right place.
> • Reduce hunting and gathering for supplies.
> • Feed forward the needed information just in time.

5. Changes → Develop Change Ideas

What ideas do we have for changing what is currently done (the process) to get better results? Use brainstorming or nominal group methods to generate a long list of change ideas. Use multivoting or another method to reduce the list to the top priorities for actual testing in a pilot study. Consider multiple sources for potential changes based on the work done to analyze outcomes (Step 1), processes (Step 2), patterns (Step 3), and structure (Step 4). Also consider developing more change ideas based on a search of the literature, best practices review and benchmarking (see Chapter 5), and the application of change concepts (see Chapter 6).

> **Tips:** Set up this task by asking group members to step back for a moment and to think about the aim, the desired results (clinical, functional, satisfaction, costs), and the delivery process, patterns, and structural characteristics which they have explored. Then, based on their own ideas and analysis (or based on another

person's or expert's ideas or analysis), ask participants to write down (silently and on their own) as many changes as they can think of which might result in better, safer care and lower costs. Ask each member to read one idea, rotating around the group to develop an exhaustive list of change ideas. Clarify these concepts and combine those which are redundant. Use multivoting, or another method, to help determine the most promising change idea for pilot testing.

6. Pilot → Select First/Next Change for Pilot Testing

How can we pilot test an improvement idea using the PDSA (Plan-Do-Study-Act) method? It's essential to know if a change results in an improvement; thus, it is wise to pilot test most proposed changes. The most common design for pilot testing is a simple before-and-after study comparing the old way with the new way. If possible, it's best to test the change quickly on a small scale using the rapid tests of change approach.[2,3] There might be logistical, political, or timing issues that support or hinder a pilot test, and these should be identified now.

> **Tips:** Not all changes will necessarily be pilot tested. Some might be "quick and easy" to accomplish, will produce obvious and immediate improvements, and thereby, obviate need for a pilot (for example, giving patients an accurate, legible written regimen can improve understanding of the treatment plan). It is sometimes possible to use a more powerful design than a simple before-and-after trial, for example, controlled trials, randomized designs, or factorial designs.[4]

Side B: Aim...Fire...Hit (Or Miss)

A. Selected Change → How Would We Describe the Change We Have Selected for Testing?

List here the most promising change ideas that came from completion of Step 5 (or that have been identified since then), and provide a general description of the change that has been selected for testing.

> **Tips:** This is a "holding pool" of potential changes to be tried out in the future. (The essence of continual improvement is to run repeated, increasingly effective, and increasingly rapid tests of changes.) It also is a place

FIGURE A-7. **Clinical Value Compass Worksheet, Side A**

OUTCOMES → Select a population _____

(specify patient population)

AIM → What's the general aim? Given our aim to limit or reduce the illness burden for "this type" of patient, what are the desired results?

VALUE → Select starter set of outcomes/cost measures

Functional & Risk Status
- Physical function
- Mental health
- Social/Role Function
- Other (eg, pain, health risk)

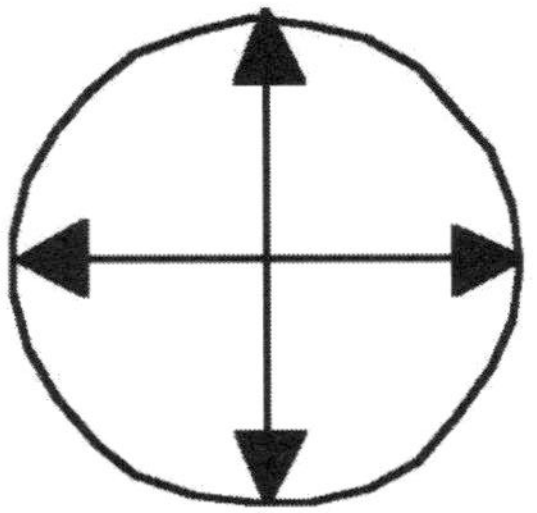

Satisfaction Against Need
- Health care delivery
- Perceived health benefit

Costs
- Direct medical
- Indirect social

Clinical Outcomes
- Mortality
- Morbidity
- Complications
- Adverse Events causing harm

TIPS: Path Forward →

Worksheet purpose : To identify measures of outcomes/costs that contribute most to the value of care.

1. Select a clinically significant population.

2. Assemble small interdisciplinary work group.

3. Use brainstorming or nominal group technique to generate "long" list of measures

4. Start with west (clinical) on the compass and go clockwise around the compass.

5. Use multivoting to identify "short" list of 4 to 12 key measures of outcomes and costs.

6. Determine what data are needed versus what data can be obtained in real time at affordable cost.

7. Use side B of worksheet to record names and definitions of selected measures of value.

FIGURE A-9. Clinical Value Compass Worksheet, Side B

SPECIFIC OPERATIONAL DEFINITIONS for key outcome and cost measures

Variable name and brief conceptual definition	Source of data and operation and definition
A. _____ Owner: _____	
B. _____ Owner: _____	
C. _____ Owner: _____	
D. _____ Owner: _____	
E. _____ Owner: _____	
F. _____ Owner: _____	
G. _____ Owner: _____	
H. _____ Owner: _____	

TIPS: Writing Definitions

A *conceptual definition* is a brief statement describing a variable of interest. It should tell people <u>what</u> you want to measure and who "owns" it.

An *operational definition* is a clearly specified <u>method</u> for reliably sorting, classifying, or measuring a variable. It should be written as an instruction set, or protocol, that would enable two different people to measure the variable, by using the same process and thereby producing the same result. It should explain to people <u>how</u> a variable should be measured.

FIGURE A-10. **Benchmarking for Best Practices, Side 1**

Aim: Develop ideas about best practices.

1. Identify measures.

Using the Clinical Value Compass as a guide, reach a consensus on 2 or 3 statistical measures, or benchmarks, that will be the focus of the external scan. Consider the availability of valid comparative data and variability of performance across facilities. (An appropriate benchmark enables measurement and comparison across systems.)

Functional Health Status

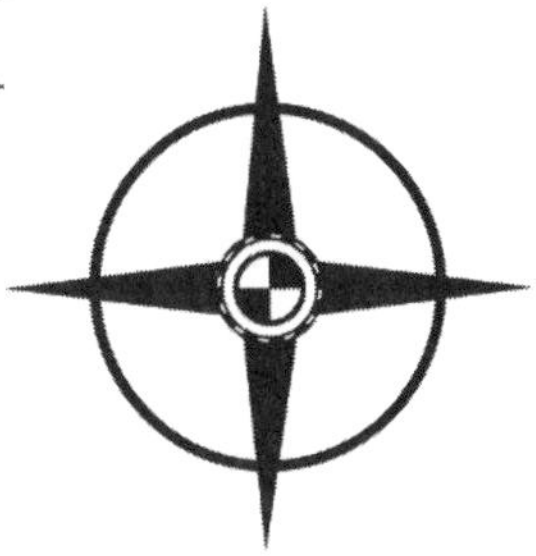

Clinical Outcomes

Satisfaction Against Need

Total Costs

2. Determine resources needed to find the best of the best.

Given our desire to limit or reduce the illness burden (cost, resource use, excess morbidity, mortality) for our patients, think about the information needed for finding the best of the best.

The best data to use? Internal? External?	The best people to ask? In-house? Out-of-house?

The best literature?

FIGURE A-11. **Benchmarking for Best Practices, Side 2**

3. **Design data-collection method and gather data.**
   Who will collect the data? How will the data be analyzed? Who will review the literature?

Task: **Person completing:**   **Date to be completed:**

_____

_____

_____

_____

_____

_____

4. **Measure best against own performance to determine gap.**
   Based on the measures identified in step 1, and the results of an internal and external scan of the data, how does our performance compare to the best of the best?

Benchmark: _____

Our results _____

Average _____

"Best" _____

Summary Data
Number of cases: _____
Total revenue: _____
Revenue rank: _____

Benchmark: _____

Our results _____

Average _____

"Best" _____

Benchmark: _____

Our results _____

Average _____

"Best" _____

Functional Health Status

Clinical Outcomes / Satisfaction Against Need

Total Costs

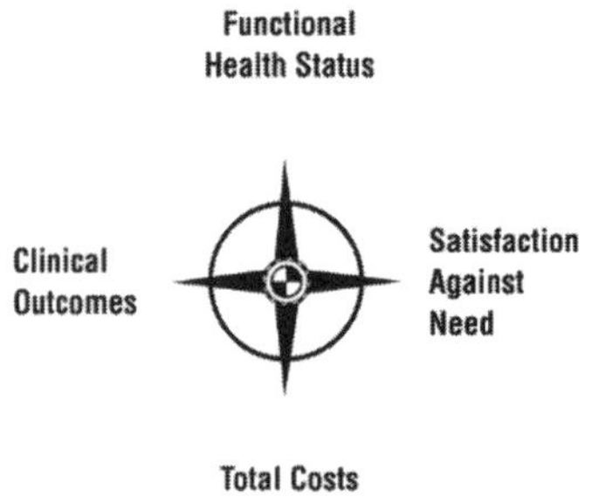

Compared to what we found, how good is our quality and value?

Benchmark: _____

Our results _____

Average _____

"Best" _____

Benchmark: _____

Our results _____

Average _____

"Best" _____

Benchmark: _____

Our results _____

Average _____

"Best" _____

5. **Identify the best practices that produce best-in-class results.**

FIGURE A-12. **A Generic Model for Making and Sustaining Improvements: PDSA ↔ SDSA Worksheet, Page 1**

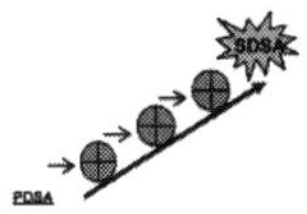

PDSA ↔ SDSA Worksheet

Name of Group: _____   Start Date:_____

TEAM MEMBERS

1. Leader: _____   5. _____
2. Facilitator: _____   6. _____
3. _____   7. _____
4. _____   8. _____

Coach: _____   Meeting Day/Time: _____

Data Support: _____   Place: _____

1. ***Aim*** ➡ What are we trying to accomplish?

2. ***Measures*** ➡ How will we know that a change is an improvement?

3. ***Current Process*** ➡ What is the process for giving care to this type of patient?

Note: Questions 1, 2, and 3 are bigger picture (30,000 feet type) questions.
        Questions 4–8 are very specific, ground-level questions.
This worksheet can be used to plan and keep track of improvement efforts.

Figure A-12. The PDSA—SDSA worksheet focuses on establishing a lead team and aim.

(continued)

FIGURE A-12. **A Generic Model for Making and Sustaining Improvements: PDSA ↔ SDSA Worksheet, Page 2**

Plan → How shall we PLAN the pilot? Who does what and when? With what tools or training?
  • Baseline data to be collected? How will we know if a change is an improvement?

Tasks to be completed to run test of change	Who	When	Tools/Training Needed	Measures

Do → What are we learning as we ***DO*** the pilot? What happened when we ran the test? Any problems encountered? Any surprises?

Study → As we ***STUDY*** what happened, what have we learned? What do the measures show?

Act → As we ***ACT*** to hold the gains or abandon our pilot efforts, what needs to be done? Will we modify the change? Make PLAN for the next cycle of change.

Standardize → Once you have determined this PDSA result to be the current "best practice" take action to Standardize-Do-Study-Act (SDSA). You will create the conditions to ensure this "best practice" in daily activities until a NEW change is identified and then the SDSA moves back to the PDSA cycle to test the idea to then standardize again.

FIGURE A-12. **A Generic Model for Making and Sustaining Improvements: PDSA ↔ SDSA Worksheet, Page 3**

Tradeoffs ➤ What are we NOT going to do anymore to support this new habit?

What has helped us in the past to change behavior and helped us do the "right thing?"

What type of environment has supported standardization?

How do we design the new "best practice" to be the default step in the process?

Consider professional behaviors, attitudes, values, and assumptions when designing how to embed this new "best practice."

Measures ➤ How will we know that this process continues to be an improvement?

What measures will inform us if "standardization" is in practice?

How will we know if "old behaviors" have appeared again?

How will we measure? How often? Who?

This worksheet can be used to plan-standardize and keep track of improvement efforts.

(continued)

FIGURE A-12. **A Generic Model for Making and Sustaining Improvements: PDSA ↔ SDSA Worksheet, Page 4**

Possible Changes → Are there identified needs for change or new information or "tested" best practice to test? What is the change idea? Who will oversee the new PDSA? Go to PDSA worksheet.

Standardize → How shall we *STANDARDIZE* the process and embed it into daily practice? Who? Does what? When? With what tools? What needs to be "unlearned" to allow this new habit? What data will inform us if this is being standardized daily?

Tasks to be completed to "embed" standardization and monitor process to run test of change	Who	When	Tools/Training Needed	Measures
*Playbook- Create standard process map to be inserted in your Playbook.				

Do → What are we learning as we *DO* the standardization? Any problems encountered? Any surprises? Any new insights to lead to another PDSA cycle?

Study → As we *STUDY* the standardization, what have we learned? What do the measures show? Are there identified needs for change or new information or "tested" best practice to adapt?

Act → As we **ACT** to hold the gains or modify the standardization efforts, what needs to be done? Will we modify the standardization? What is the change idea? Who will oversee the new PDSA? Design new PDSA cycle. Make PLAN for the next cycle of change. Go to PDSA worksheet.

to record a brief description of the selected change before proceeding to a detailed plan.

B. Aim → What Are We Trying to Accomplish (More Specific Aim)?

Make a more specific aim statement that is in line with the original, general aim statement and that serves as a clear objective for the proposed pilot. In the process of converting the general aim into a more specific aim, sharpen the objective by taking into consideration the relevant aspects of structure, process, and pattern.

> **Tips:** A structured aim statement is often helpful. For example: "An opportunity exists to improve [name the process]. The process starts when [insert start point] and ends when [insert end point]. It is expected that improvement in this process will [insert likely improvements in outcomes/costs]. It is important to work on this process now because [state clinical/business/ learning need for selecting this process now]."

An example of a structured aim follows. An opportunity exists to improve the process of diagnosing patients who come to our emergency department. The process starts when a patient enters the emergency room and reports to the receptionist. The process ends when the clinician makes a diagnosis or establishes the problem to be treated. It is expected that improvement in this process will (a) increase the timeliness of the assessment process, (b) decrease the amount of time the patient spends in the emergency department, and (c) increase patient satisfaction with the care they receive in the emergency department. It is important to work on this now because many patients have complained about how long they have had to wait before receiving care and some clinical quality measures show that the waiting time before the start of treatment often exceeds national standards of care.

C. Measures → How Will We Know Whether a Change Is an Improvement?

Select one or two primary outcome measures that can be used to evaluate the success (outcomes and costs) of the pilot test. Consider using a countermeasure to detect unwanted side effects.

> **Tips:** Measures should flow from the specific aim statement cited in Step A and from the more

general, higher-level list of outcomes/costs that came from Step 1. It is often wise to:
- Include fewer rather than more measures to avoid data overload.
- Select a few patient descriptors to characterize case mix, a few process measures to indicate how process is changing or staying the same, and a small balanced set of measures of quality and costs.

D. Plan → How Shall We Plan the Pilot?

Who? Does what? When? With what tools and training? Write a brief change protocol that answers these questions. Illustrate the protocol with a simple flowchart.

> **Tips:** A good plan must be executed well to succeed. This means that all involved should know what they are doing and why they are doing it. Writing down the specifics in black and white and illustrating these steps with a flowchart is a good start. Discuss the plan with all those who will be executing it; be prepared to make refinements and changes as needed.

Baseline data to be collected? Write a brief data collection protocol indicating who will gather and analyze what data from what sources based on operational definitions.

> **Tips:** Specify the key questions to be answered by the pilot test, and create a "dummy" version of how data will be displayed to answer these key questions. A dummy data display is a make-believe table or data display that shows exactly how the data will be analyzed and summarized. It often takes the form of a graphical data display showing changes over time using a run chart or control chart and/or a data table showing results before and after a change is made. Include the operational definitions to be used for each variable in the data collection plan. Whenever possible, build the data collection into the flow of the work; design "self-coding" data collection forms that can be used by people as care is delivered. Often a pocket-sized, preprinted card can be used to gather values on variables that are not routinely or accurately recorded in normal clinical or administrative databases. (Note: Chapter 4, which addresses measuring outcomes and

costs, contains more information and a worksheet for operational definitions.)

E. Do → What Are We Learning as We Do the Pilot? (structure, process, pattern)

Keep a diary of the pilot test. Jot down notes on how the pilot is going, including information on whether all steps are proceeding as planned. Reflect on what is working or failing, and consider the significance of any surprises that might occur.

> **Tips:** Improvement work is full of unanticipated events that might positively or negatively influence the results of the pilot. Also, the results of the pilot will be no better than the care with which the planned change is executed. Observations on the process of change can prepare the way for making bigger, more powerful changes in future.

F. Study → As We Study and Check What Happened, What Have We Learned? (structure, process, pattern)

Did original outcomes improve? Analyze the results of the pilot test of change in a way that answers the main question: Did the change lead to the predicted improvement? Were there any unanticipated effects? Were these effects constructive or destructive?

> **Tips:** Consider summarizing the key results graphically and leading off each graph with a question that is answered by the data display. One method of summarizing the results (that links case mix with process changes with outcomes and cost results) is to place before-and-after measures on key points in the process outcome flowchart. This creates a process-based instrument panel.[5–7]

G. Act → As We Act to Hold the Gains or Abandon Our Pilot Efforts, What Needs to Be Done? (structure, process, pattern)

If the pilot was successful, and if it was performed on a small scale or a temporary basis, determine what next steps are required to efficiently and effectively build the successful change into daily work routines. Make a plan for mainstreaming the change into daily work and begin to implement it. If the pilot was unsuccessful, analyze the source(s) of the failure. Was this due to a change concept that did not work or a change concept that was not prop-

erly implemented? If the former is more likely to be true, then consider going back to the "holding pool" of promising changes and select another for a pilot test.

> **Tips:** Many tests of change fail to produce the desired results. Do not be discouraged; much can be learned from failures. Use this new knowledge to feed into more effective, next-phase change attempts.

H. SDSA (Standardize-Do-Study-Act) → How Do We Ensure That Changes Are Standardized and Practiced?

It is very common for a change effort to lead to an initial improvement that is lost over time. It is well known that it is easier to make improvements than to make sustained improvements. The question is: How do we hold the gains until further improvements or innovations are made? A good approach to prevent the deterioration of improvement is to recognize the value of "oscillatons" between testing changes (i.e., being in a PDSA mode, which involves experimentation) and sustaining changes (i.e., being in a SDSA mode, which involves standardization).

> **Tips:** Prepare a flowchart to graphically illustrate who does what, when, and in what sequence. This process map can then be used: (1) to teach people how to carry out the process in a standard, best-known way; (2) to check actual work routines against the standard routine to promote follow-through and accountability; and (3) to serve as the "current process" against which new pilot test processes are compared when switching back over to PDSA mode.

What do we measure and monitor over time?

One reason that improvements degrade over time is that people's attention shifts to other matters; there are no reminders nor any way to know that performance is deteriorating. A powerful antidote to this common problem is to use some key measure(s) to monitor performance over time. This is the value of having a valuable, useful, and used "dashboard" or "instrument panel" that offers constant and visual feedback on how things are working.

> **Tips:** Construct a "data wall" to serve as a "dashboard" that monitors key performance indicators. Review and discuss the dashboard metrics on a regular basis with all the members

of the microsystem who are engaged in the process and who therefore contribute to the outcomes. A visually rich information environment is a powerful trigger to action. If dashboard measures are staying in the "right zone," this suggests that the new process is continuing to function correctly. If metrics decline (rapidly or gradually) or if they vary widely, "upstream" or underlying conditions might have changed, in which case further improvements must be considered. Alternatively, conditions have remained stable, and the initial improvement is still viable, but retraining of staff is required.

Side C: Ready...Flowchart of Basic Clinical Process

Side C (Figure A-5, page 141) provides a conceptual overview and work space for creating a flowchart of the basic clinical process. Basic tips on flowchart creation are also provided.

Side D: Ready...Measurement of Key a Variable

Side D (Figure A-6, page 142) provides a worksheet for construction of a statistical process control chart to track a primary measure of process performance. As reviewed sequentially on the worksheet, creation of an XMR-style control chart proceeds in three basic steps:

- Step 1 involves entering the data.
- Step 2 requires calculations based on these data; necessary formulas are listed in the second tier of the worksheet.
- Step 3 entails plotting of data over time while showing statistical process control limits and averages.

The XMR control chart is among the most powerful and commonly utilized display instruments. It is a flexible and robust method for demonstrating longitudinal trends in data, including measures (variables) based on counts (for example, number of people seen per day with elevated diastolic blood pressure), on rates (for example, number of people per 100 seen with elevated diastolic blood pressure), or on averages of repeated small samples (for example, average diastolic blood pressure of consecutive patients seen over time in subsample groupings of five each). For more information on XMR control charts refer to introductory texts.[8,9]

References

1. Scholtes P., Joiner B., Streibel B.: *The Team Handbook,* 2nd ed. Madison, WI: Oriel, Inc., 2000.
2. Institute for Healthcare Improvement: *Home Page.* http://www.IHI.org (accessed Jan. 27, 2007).
3. Langley G.J., et al.: *The Improvement Guide: A Practical Approach to Enhancing Organizational Performance.* San Francisco: Jossey-Bass Publishers, 1996.
4. Nelson E.C., et al.: Good measurement for good improvement work. *Qual Manag Health Care* 13:1–16, Jan.–Mar. 2004.
5. Nelson E., et al.: Report cards or instrument panels: Who needs what? *Jt Comm J Qual Improv* 21:155–166, Apr. 1995.
6. Nelson E.C., Batalden P.B.: Patient-based quality measurement systems. *Qual Manag Health Care* 2:18–30, Fall 1993.
7. Nugent W.C., et al.: Designing an instrument panel to monitor and improve coronary artery bypass grafting. *Journal of Clinical Outcomes Management* 1:57–64, Dec. 1994.
8. Carey R.G., Lloyd R.C.: *Measuring Quality Improvement in Healthcare: A Guide to Statistical Process Control Applications.* New York City: Quality Resources, 1995.
9. Wheeler D.J.: *Understanding Variation: The Key to Managing Chaos.* Knoxville, TN: SPC Press, 1993.

QUALITATIVE METHODS: OBSERVATIONAL AND INTERVIEWING WORKSHEETS

Eugene C. Nelson, Marjorie M. Godfrey

Gaining Knowledge of Patients Using Direct Observations and Individual Interviews

Introduction

The ultimate aim of improvement in health care is to find better and better ways to meet the patient's and family's needs and thereby to decrease the burden of illness and increase the level of wellness experienced by the patient and family.

The focus of this Appendix is on the phrase "experienced by the patient and family." An excellent way to launch clinical improvement work is by doing, in a planned way, what we do all the time—observe people and talk with people. These techniques are often referred to as "observations" and "interviews," and they can be used to gain insight into the way things really work—which drives outcomes—and into the perceptions of patients and families about the quality of the care that they receive—which drives satisfaction and loyalty.[1]

No methods for understanding what to do to improve care in a particular health care setting are more powerful than using observations and interviews. There are different ways to conduct observations and interviews, such as the following:

- Participant observation: taking part in care delivery and reflecting on what is seen, heard, and felt
- Direct observation: looking in on actual (or simulated) care being delivered and analyzing the process to detect inefficiency, unreliability, and unsafe practices and working conditions
- Individual interviews: conducting a focused conversation with individual patients and individual family members to gain deep insight into how they perceive their health and their experiences in receiving health care

Participant Observation: A Way to Reveal the Patients' Perceptions of Their Experience

One powerful observational technique is to set up situations that enable one to experience (see, hear, talk, feel) patients' health care journeys as they do, that is to, "walk in their shoes." Using the worksheet Through the Eyes of Your Patients (Figure B-1, page 158) provides an opportunity to see the journey—the visit to the office, the visit to the emergency department, the time spent in an inpatient care unit, the home visit by a visiting nurse—from the patient and family perspective. This technique uses role playing to simulate the experiences of being a patient (or a family member of a patient) with a certain health condition receiving care in a specific context. Through the Eyes of Your Patients offers simple guidance for using this powerful observational method. It is especially useful to gain a better understanding of the patient's and family's subjective impressions (their perceptions) about how they are being treated, which shapes people's evaluation of the quality of the care that they receive.

Direct Observation: A Way to Uncover Waste, Rework, Unreliability, and Threats to Safety and Reliability

Another powerful observational technique used extensively in many of the most successful and improvement-oriented organizations in the world (such as Toyota) is direct observation of the "real work." Improvement often starts with careful observation and reflection on how things are done in the real world under normal operating conditions. Does the process include unnecessary effort, rework, extra steps, work-arounds, unreliable features, potential safety threats, or waste of any kind (motion, resources, and so on)? These observations can generate a deep and accurate understanding of the processes and can be used to identify process imperfections associated with waste, rework, unreliability, and threats to safety. The Clinical Microsystem Observation Worksheet (Figure B-2, page 159)

FIGURE B-1. **Through the Eyes of Your Patients: A Guide to Conducting a Patient-Experience Simulation of Care**

Patients

Aim: Gain insight into how your patients experience the process of interacting with clinical services. One simple way to understand both patient flow and patient perceptions of receiving care is to experience the care through the eyes of a patient. Members of your staff can do a simulated care experience by "walking through" the care experience using role playing to simulate care delivery. Try to make this experience as real as possible; this form can be used to document the experience. You can also capture the patient experience by making an audio or videotape.

Through the Eyes of Your Patients

Tips for making the "walk through" most productive:

1. Determine with your staff where the starting point and ending points should be, taking into consideration appointment making or entering the clinical system, admissions, the actual office visit or clinical care process, follow-up, and other issues you may suspect are problems.
2. Two members of the staff should do the walk through together if possible, with each playing a role: patient and partner/family member.
3. Set aside a reasonable amount of time to experience the patient journey. Consider the usual amount of time patients spend in your clinic or in your clinical unit.

4. Make it real. Have a real appointment with a real clinician or a real visit to an emergency department, or other typical process of being admitted or discharged from an inpatient unit. Include time with lab tests, and arranging for reports to be delivered. Sit where the patient sits, lie where the patient lies. Wear what the patient wears. Make a realistic paper trail including chart, lab reports, discharge planning, and payment arrangements.
5. During the walk-through note both positive and negative experiences, as well as any surprises. What was frustrating? What was gratifying? What was confusing? Again, an audio or video tape can be helpful.
6. Debrief your staff on what you did and what you learned.

Date: _____   Staff Members: _____

Walk Through Begins When: _____   Ends When: _____

Positives	Negatives	Surprises	Frustrating/Confusing	Gratifying

FIGURE B-2. **Clinical Microsystem Observation Worksheet**

CONTEXT

Aim: Build customer knowledge through observation

① Outcomes ➞ select a patient population

(Specify patient population)

② Aim ➞ What's the general aim? Given our wish to limit or reduce the illness burden for "this type" of patient, what are the desired results?
Structured Aim Statement ➞ We aim to improve the
for

(Insert process name)   *(Insert patient population name)*

(Insert start of process boundary)

(Insert end of process boundary)

By working on this process we hope to achieve these benefits:

(List benefits)

It is important to work on this process now because:

(List compelling reasons)

③ Microsystems ➞ Given the process boundaries, the clinical microsystem(s) that serve this patient population for this process are:

(List microsystem(s) serving patients)

Observation # _____ : **Facts**

Today's Date:
Patient Name/Initials:
Family Member Name/Initials:
Microsystem Name:
Provider Name/Initials:
Permission Obtained:
Time Observation Started:
Time Observation Ended:
Name of Process Observed:

Tips. Process Observation *(Watch and listen for)*

Who did what when?
What did the patient want?
What did the patient need?
Did anything delight the patient?

Did anything disappoint or upset the patient?
Did the patient experience any problems?
What was the patient saying? Thinking?
What did "body language" say?

④ Observer: _____ Date: _____

Person being observed: _____

Observation begins with: _____

Activities Observed

When	Where	What	Who	Saying What

Observation ends with: _____

© 2003, Trustees of Dartmouth College, Nelson, Godfrey: Rev. 05/10/03

FIGURE B-3. **The Clinical Microsystem Interview Worksheet**

Tips

1. Eye contact
2. Comfortable environment
3. Consider audio/video taping
4. Follow clues... eg "High quality... what would that look like? How would you describe quality?"
5. Observe body language and facial expressions

Note Taking Tips

1. Discuss note taking with interviewee
2. Take notes regularly and promptly
3. Try "close" to verbatim note taking
4. Don't let note taking interfere with ability to listen and ask questions

Steps of an Individual Interview

- Preflight
  - Review your aim and interview guide.
- Taking Off
  - Establish purpose with respondent and rapport and appreciation for their participation.
- Flying
  - Work your way through the interview guide covering the main topics, exploring promising leads, and asking questions to clarify and to probe.
- Landing
  - Ask your final question, remind the respondent of how results will be used, and thank him for participating.
- Debriefing
  - Reflect on how the interview went
  - What might be done to improve the process and the method before conducting the next interview

Interview # _____ : Facts

Today's Date:
Patient Name/Initials:
Family Member Name/Initials:
Microsystem Name:
Provider Name/Initials:
Permission Obtained:
Time Interview Started:
Time Interview Ended:
Aim of Interview:

Steps for Doing Interviews

1. **Aim.** Set the aim and frame the key question(s).
2. **Who.** Determine who will be interviewed and how they will be invited to participate.
3. **Plan.** Who will conduct the interviews, in what setting and with what tools and training? How will the results be recorded and analyzed?
4. **Interviews.** Conduct the interviews using an interview guide.
5. **Analysis.** Analyze the content of the results to identify the response patterns that provide answers to your key question(s).
6. **Summarize.** Reflect on you analysis and summarize the results. Consider doing this by using "major results" that are linked to actual verbatim statement contained in the interview notes.

FIGURE B-3. (continued)
The Clinical Microsystem Interview Worksheet

Interview Guide Template

<u>Preflight</u>
- Interview who, where, under what auspices, with what guide, for what purpose

<u>Taking Off</u>
- Introduce self, purpose of interview, how information is to be used, assure confidentiality, ask any questions and ask permission to proceed with the interview.
- First question . . . Write an open-ended question that invites the respondent to tell his/her "story" re: topic of interest . . .

My first question is: _____

<u>Flying</u>
- Frame several "core" questions to achieve your aim and answer key questions.
  1. _____
  2. _____
  3. _____
  4. _____
  5. _____

<u>Landing</u>
- Last question . . . Write summative last question. . .

My last question is: _____

- Thank respondent and say goodbye.

<u>Debriefing</u>
- If taking notes . . . Review notes and add to them to make as complete a record as possible
- Consider what new is learned by this interview
- Consider refinements to interview guide based on what was learned

© 2003, Trustees of Dartmouth College, Nelson, Godfrey: Rev. 05/10/03

(continued)

FIGURE B-3. (continued)
The Clinical Microsystem Interview Worksheet

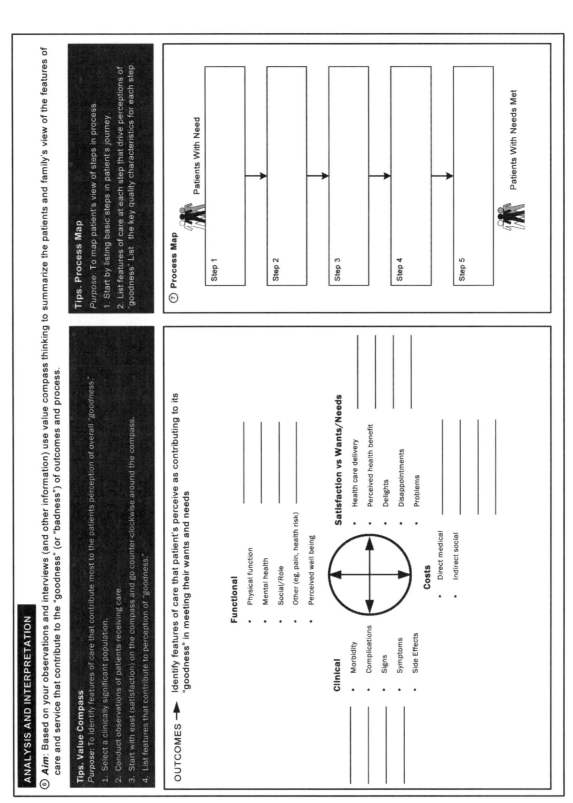

provides a method for documenting process flows —the way things work—on the basis of the observed patient experience in a specific clinical context.

For a more elaborate approach to work flow observation, a useful technique is value stream mapping, a sophisticated, detailed process analysis method that includes both the sequence of actions and the flow of information that is associated with the actions.[2,3]

Individual Interviews: A Way to Learn About Perceptions on Being Cared For and Receiving Care

Individual interviews offer another powerful and flexible method for gaining knowledge about the patient's and family's perceptions of their experiences in health care, and about their interactions with physicians, nurses, and other staff. Holding a special, private conversation with a patient—or with a family member who is part of that patient's support system—can produce a rich bounty of stories, insights, and impressions that are perceived as important aspects of the process of caring, the nature of the relationships, and the perceived benefits stemming from the health care received. The Clinical Microsystem Interview Worksheet (Figure B-3, pages 160–162) provides a path for planning and conducting individual interviews.

Another well-known approach for gaining qualitative information is to use focus group interviewing methods.[4,5] This is a flexible and powerful method but requires greater expertise and more detailed planning and logistics than individual, in-depth interviews.

Observing the "Real Work" of Clinical Care

The plastic surgery section at Dartmouth-Hitchcock Medical Center has been actively engaged in efforts to improve local care. Team members have worked toward the interdependent goals of optimizing patient outcomes and (through elimination of waste and rework in the process of care) creating a more joyful work experience for clinicians and staff themselves. The use of observation techniques has been extremely beneficial to the improvement effort.

In the endoscopic surgical treatment of carpal tunnel syndrome, for example, videotaping of the entire procedure has led to significant improvements in perioperative surgical care processes. Review of videotapes, which include all interventions from initial setup to final cleanup, has enabled team members to see many opportunities for improvement that were previously hidden, including elimination of waste and reduction in unnecessary variation.

The advantage of videotaping is that *all* members of a practice team can visualize current processes as these occur in the real world. This visualization promotes recognition of specific improvement opportunities, and facilitates buy-in of all participants, who can then work together to modify activities and eliminate waste. For the plastic surgery team, the videotape highlighted variation between two registered nurses who assisted the surgeon on different days, resulting in highly varied processes. When the lead improvement team reviewed the videotape, it was able to create process maps and to highlight "best practices;" the nurses were then empowered to standardize the process, resulting in benefit to both patients and staff.

This new standardization enabled the surgeon to increase her productivity from 3–4 carpal tunnel procedures to 6–8 procedures per session. At the same time, specific responsibilities in the care process could be matched more effectively to specific team members on the basis of education, training, and licensure, thereby freeing time for the surgeon and nurse to engage in other appropriate activities within the practice. Finally, the group was able to build standard carpal tunnel kits and to decrease the number of surgical packs from six to two; procedures for setup and cleanup were standardized as well. Because of these and other new efficiencies, the same practice has more recently been able to run two procedure rooms at the same time, greatly enhancing productivity with no reduction in quality of care.

References

1. Lee F.: *If Disney Ran Your Hospital: 9 1/2 Things You Would Do Differently.* Bozeman, MT: Second River Healthcare, 2004.
2. George M., et al.: *The Lean Six Sigma Pocket Toolbook.* New York City: McGraw Hill, 2005.
3. Rother, M., Shook H.: *Learning to See: Value Stream Mapping to Create Value and Eliminate Muda,* version 1.1. 1998. Cambridge, MA: The Lean Enterprise Institute.
4. Morgan D.L., Krueger R.A. (eds.): *The Focus Group Kit,* vols 1–6. Thousand Oaks, CA: Sage Publications, 1998.
5. Stewart D., Shamdasani P.: *Focus Groups: Theory and Practice.* Applied Social Research Methods Series. Newbury Park, CA: Sage Publications, Inc., 1990.

Patient-Reported Measures of Quality and Value

Eugene C. Nelson

Methods for measuring quality and value are advancing rapidly ,and their use is proliferating. Policy makers, researchers, practitioners, payers, and patients are increasingly vocal in their demand for better measures of quality and costs. Clinical Value Compass thinking provides a practical model for connecting a balanced set of outcomes, reflecting both quality and cost, with the process of care that produces these results.

One obstacle to measuring quality and value is lack of availability of—or knowledge of—practical, validated measures that can be used in, or adapted to, real-world clinical settings. For more detailed information on quality and value measurement, please refer to the extensive and important body of published work, including the Institute of Medicine's *Performance Measurement: Accelerating Improvement*[1]; the large series of reports and publications that have been distributed by the National Quality Forum[2]; the quality metrics proposed by the Agency for Healthcare Research and Quality (AHRQ), Quality Indicators[3]; the cost and quality measures used in the Dartmouth Atlas of Health Care[4]; and the Institute for Healthcare Improvement's useful work on measures of health system performance known as Whole System Measures.[5]

Although a detailed compendium of validated quality and value measures is well beyond the scope of this book, we offer here some representative, patient-based measures that can be used for practice-based learning and improvement. Given the ongoing trend toward customized, patient-centered, preference-sensitive care, patient surveys such as these are valuable sources of primary data on quality and cost.

The measures in this appendix have been selected because they are patient-based (or patient family–based) and because they meet the following criteria:

- Practical utility for large groups of patients
- Adaptable for widespread use in busy health care settings
- Rigorously tested to establish relevance, reliability, and validity

The surveys included in this appendix cover three different topics:

- To measure clinical and health statuses of patients or community residents, consider using one of the eight "clinical and health status surveys."
- To measure patients' viewpoints and perceptions about the quality of their health care, consider using one of the four "patient satisfaction and perceptions surveys."
- To get a sense of the kinds and amounts of health care that patients are using, consider using the "patient utilization question survey."

References

1. Institute of Medicine: *Performance Measurement: Accelerating Improvement.* Washington, DC: National Academy Press, 2006.
2. National Quality Forum (NQF): *National Priorities for Healthcare Quality Measurement and Reporting.* Washington, D.C.: NQF, 2004.
3. Agency for Healthcare Research and Quality (AHRQ): *General Questions About the AHRQ Quality Indicators.* http://www.qualityindicators.ahrq.gov/general_faq.htm#1 (accessed Jun. 4, 2007).
4. The Dartmouth Atlas Project: *The Dartmouth Atlas of Health Care.* http://www.dartmouthatlas.org (accessed Jun. 4, 2007).
5. Lloyd R., Martin L., Nelson E.: *IHI's Whole System Measures Tool Kit: Version 2.0.* Institute for Healthcare Improvement, Jul. 18, 2006. http://www.ihi.org/NR/rdonlyres/0848B270-EA39-4B90-9AC2-2C8DF3A1379D/3644/IHIWholeSystemMeasuresToolkitV271906.pdf (accessed Jun. 4, 2007).

Chronic Conditions Checklist

Source: Eugene C. Nelson, Dartmouth Medical School, 1997. Adapted from the Medical Outcomes Study, The Rand Corporation, 1986. Used with permission.

Has a doctor <u>ever</u> told you that you had:	Yes	No
1. Hypertension or high blood pressure	☐	☐
2. Angina pectoris or coronary artery disease (CAD)	☐	☐
3. Congestive heart failure or an enlarged heart	☐	☐
4. A myocardial infarction or heart attack	☐	☐
5. Other heart conditions, such as problems with heart valves or the rhythm of your heartbeat	☐	☐
6. A stroke	☐	☐
7. Emphysema, asthma, or COPD (chronic obstructive pulmonary disease)	☐	☐
8. Crohn's disease, ulcerative colitis, or inflammatory bowel disease	☐	☐
9. An ulcer or other disorder of the gastrointestinal tract	☐	☐
10. Arthritis of the hip or knee	☐	☐
11. Arthritis of any other joint	☐	☐
12. Osteoporosis	☐	☐
13. Diabetes, high blood sugar, or sugar in your urine	☐	☐
14. Non-malignant tumor or growth	☐	☐
15. Cancer (diagnosed in the last 3 years, except skin cancer)	☐	☐
16. Kidney disease	☐	☐

Are you <u>currently under treatment</u> for:	Yes	No
17. Cancer of any kind	☐	☐
18. Kidney dialysis	☐	☐

Do you <u>now have</u>:	Yes	No
19. A regular or daily cough	☐	☐
20. Shortness of breath when walking less than 1 block	☐	☐
21. Acid indigestion or heartburn	☐	☐
22. Trouble hearing (even with a hearing aid)	☐	☐

	Yes	**No**
23. Trouble seeing (even with glasses or contact lenses)	☐	☐

Emotional Health

24. In the *past year,* have you had *2 weeks or more* during which you felt sad, blue, or depressed; or when you lost all interest or pleasure in things that you usually care about or enjoy?   ☐ ☐

25. Have you had *2 years or more* in your life when you felt depressed or sad *most days,* even if you felt okay sometimes?   ☐ ☐

Dartmouth Primary Care Cooperative Research Network (COOP) Charts: Adults

Sourse: Wasson JH, et. al., and the trustees of Dartmouth College/COOP Project (Lebanon, NH), © 1989. Used with permission.

SOCIAL ACTIVITIES

During the past 4 weeks . . .
  Has your physical and emotional health limited your social activities with family, friends, neighbors or groups?

Not at all		**1**
Slightly		**2**
Moderately		**3**
Quite a bit		**4**
Extremely		**5**

PAIN

During the past 4 weeks . . .
How much bodily pain have you
generally had?

No pain		**1**
Very mild pain		**2**
Mild pain		**3**
Moderate pain		**4**
Severe pain		**5**

PHYSICAL FITNESS

During the past 4 weeks . . .
What was the hardest physical activity
you could do for at least 2 minutes?

Very heavy, (for example)
• Run, fast pace
• Carry a heavy load
  upstairs or uphill
  (25 lbs/10 kgs)
		1

Heavy, (for example) • Jog, slow pace • Climb stairs or a hill moderate pace		**2**

Moderate, (for example)
• Walk, medium pace
• Carry a heavy load
  on level ground
  (25 lbs/10 kgs)
		3

Light, (for example)
• Walk, medium pace
• Carry light load
  on level ground
  (10 lbs/5 kgs)
		4

Very light, (for example) • Walk, slow pace • Wash dishes		**5**

FEELINGS

During the past 4 weeks . . .
How much have you been bothered by
emotional problems such as feeling anxious,
depressed, irritable or downhearted and blue?

Not at all		**1**
Slightly		**2**
Moderately		**3**
Quite a bit		**4**
Extremely		**5**

DAILY ACTIVITIES

During the past 4 weeks . . .
   How much difficulty have you had doing your usual activities or task, both inside and outside the house, because of your physical and emotional health?

No difficulty at all		1
A little bit of difficulty		2
Some difficulty		3
Much difficulty		4
Could not do		5

CHANGE IN HEALTH

How would you rate your overall health now compared to 4 weeks ago?

Much better	▲▲ ++	1
A little better	▲ +	2
About the same	◄► =	3
A little worse	▼ —	4
Much worse	▼▼ ——	5

OVERALL HEALTH

During the past 4 weeks . . .
How would you rate your health in general?

Excellent		**1**
Very good		**2**
Good		**3**
Fair		**4**
Poor		**5**

SOCIAL SUPPORT

During the past 4 weeks . . .

Was someone available to help you if you
needed and wanted help? For example if you

- felt very nervous, lonely, or blue
- got sick and had to stay in bed
- needed someone to talk to
- needed help with daily chores
- needed help just taking care of yourself

Yes, as much as I wanted		**1**
Yes, quite a bit		**2**
Yes, some		**3**
Yes, a little		**4**
No, not at all		**5**

QUALITY OF LIFE

How have things been going for you during the past 4 weeks?

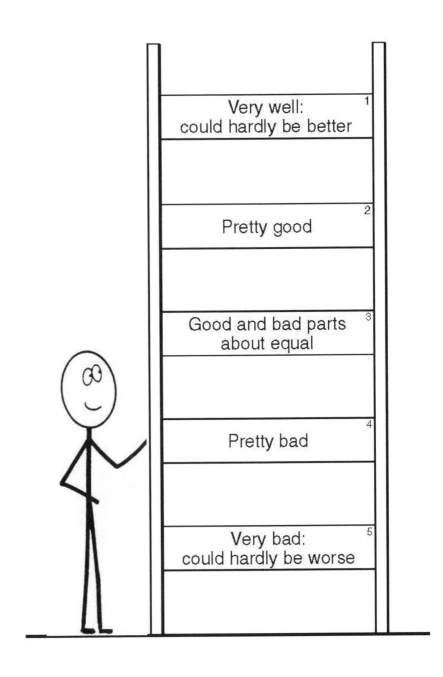

Dartmouth Primary Care Cooperative Research Network (COOP) Charts: Adolescents

PHYSICAL FITNESS

During the past month, what was the hardest physical activity you could do for <u>at least 10 minutes</u>?

Very heavy (Run, fast pace)		**1**
Heavy (Jog, slow pace)		**2**
Moderate (Walk, fast pace)		**3**
Light (Walk, regular pace)		**4**
Very Light (Walk, slow pace)		**5**

EMOTIONAL FEELINGS

During the past month, how often did you feel
anxious, depressed, irritable, sad or downhearted
and blue?

None of the time		1
A little of the time		2
Some of the time		3
Most of the time		4
All of the time		5

SCHOOL WORK

During the last month you were in school, how did you do?

I did very well		1
I did as well as I could		2
I could have done <u>a little</u>		3
better		4
I could have done <u>much</u>		5

SOCIAL SUPPORT

During the past month, if you needed someone to listen

Yes, as much as I wanted		**1**
Yes, quite a bit		**2**
Yes, some		**3**
Yes, a little		**4**
No, not at all		**5**

HEALTH HABITS I

During the past month, how often did you do things that are harmful to your health such as:
• smoke cigarettes or chew tobacco
• have unprotected sex
• use alcohol including beer or wine?

None of the time		**1**
A little of the time		**2**
Some of the time		**3**
Most of the time		**4**
All of the time		**5**

FAMILY

During the past month, how often did you talk about your problems, feelings or opinions with someone in your family?

All of the time		1
Most of the time		2
Some of the time		3
A little of the time		4
None of the time		5

Functional Health Status 6-Item Survey

Source: William H. Rogers, New England Medical Center, 2002. Adapted from the Medical Outcomes Study. Used with permission.

Patient Questionnaire

Thank you for filling out this questionnaire.

The purpose of this survey is to try to find a good way to collect information on the overall health of patients who receive care here. Your health care provider may or may not use your answers during your visit.

Instructions:
1. Please start right away and fill out as much as you can <u>before</u> your visit.
2. When you are finished, give it to your health care provider at the beginning of your visit with him/her.
3. If you do not have time to complete it before seeing your health care provider, please take a few minutes to complete it before leaving the office and give it to the receptionist.

****

Your Physical Health: The first questions ask about your physical health and activities.

1. During the past 4 weeks, how much has your health limited you in doing <u>moderate activities</u>, such as moving a table, pushing a vacuum cleaner, or walking a few blocks? Would you say you have been…

    <1> Limited a lot
    <2> Limited a little
    <3> Not limited at all

2. During the past 4 weeks, how much has your health limited you in doing <u>vigorous activities</u> such as <u>climbing several flights of stairs, lifting heavy objects, or doing strenuous sports</u>? Would you say you have been…

    <1> Limited a lot
    <2> Limited a little
    <3> Not limited at all

3. During the past 4 weeks, how much has pain <u>interfered</u> with your normal work (including both work outside the home and housework)?

      <1> Not at all
      <2> Slightly
      <3> Moderately
      <4> Quite a bit
      <5> Extremely

Your Feelings: The next questions ask about your emotional health.

4. During the past 4 weeks, how much of the time have you been <u>very nervous</u>?

      <1> All of the time
      <2> Most of the time
      <3> A good bit of the time
      <4> Some of the time
      <5> A little of the time
      <6> None of the time

5. During the past 4 weeks, how much of the time have you had a <u>lot of energy</u>?

      <1> All of the time
      <2> Most of the time
      <3> A good bit of the time
      <4> Some of the time
      <5> A little of the time
      <6> None of the time

6. During the past 4 weeks, how much of the time have you felt <u>downhearted and blue</u>?

      <1> All of the time
      <2> Most of the time
      <3> A good bit of the time
      <4> Some of the time
      <5> A little of the time
      <6> None of the time

How's your Health?

A Simple survey designed to help adults manage their health...

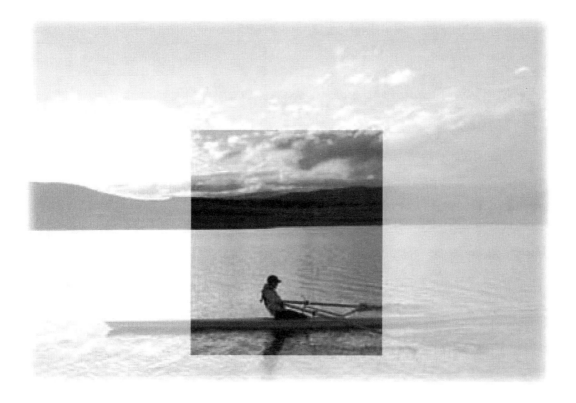

Source: John H. Wasson, FNX (Corporation under license with Trustees of Dartmouth College). The Web version of the survey is available to patients for free at http://www.howsyourhealth.org. Used with permission.

Medical Outcomes Study 12-Item Short-Form (SF-12) Health Survey

---

SF-12 HEALTH SURVEY (STANDARD)

INSTRUCTIONS: This questionnaire asks for your views about your health. This information will help keep track of how you feel and how well you are able to do your usual activities.

Please answer every question by marking one box. If you are unsure about how to answer, please give the best answer you can.

1. In general, would you say your health is:

    ☐   ☐   ☐   ☐   ☐
    Excellent   **Very Good**   **Good**   **Fair**   **Poor**

The following items are about activities you might do during a typical day. Does <u>your health now limit you</u> in these activities? If so, how much?

		Yes, Limited a Lot	Yes, Limited a Little	No, Not Limited at All
2.	**Moderate activities,** such as moving a table, pushing a vacuum cleaner, bowling, or playing golf	☐	☐	☐
3.	Climbing **several** flights of stairs	☐	☐	☐

During the <u>past 4 weeks</u>, have you had any of the following problems with your work or other regular daily activities <u>as a result of your physical health</u>?

		YES	NO
4.	**Accomplished less** than you would like	☐	☐
5.	Were limited in the **kind** of work or other activities	☐	☐

During the past 4 weeks, have you had any of the following problems with your work or other regular daily activities as a result of any emotional problems (such as feeling depressed or anxious)?

		YES	NO
6.	**Accomplished less** than you would like	☐	☐
7.	Didn't do work or other activities as **carefully** as usual	☐	☐

8. During the past 4 weeks, how much did pain interfere with your normal work (including both work outside the home and housework)?

☐	☐	☐	☐	☐
Not at All	**A Little Bit**	**Moderately**	**Quite a Bit**	**Extremely**

These questions are about how you feel and how things have been with you during the past 4 weeks. For each question, please give the one answer that comes closest to the way you have been feeling. How much of the time during the past 4 weeks -

	All of the Time	Most of the Time	A Good Bit of the Time	Some of the Time	A Little of the Time	None of the Time
9. Have you felt calm and peaceful?	☐	☐	☐	☐	☐	☐
10. Did you have a lot of energy?	☐	☐	☐	☐	☐	☐
11. Have you felt downhearted and blue?	☐	☐	☐	☐	☐	☐

12. During the past 4 weeks, how much of the time has your physical health or emotional problems interfered with your social activities (like visiting with friends, relatives, etc)?

☐	☐	☐	☐	☐
All of the Time	**Most of the Time**	**Some of the Time**	**A Little of the Time**	**None of the Time**

Medical Outcomes Study 36-Item Short-Form (SF-36) Health Survey

Source: SF-36™ and SF-12™ Health Survey, Copyright © 1992 Medical Outcomes Trust. All rights reserved. Reproduced with permission of the Medical Outcomes Trust, Boston, Massachusetts.

THE MOS 36-ITEM SHORT FORM HEALTH SURVEY (SF-36)

INSTRUCTIONS: This survey asks for your views about your health. This information will help keep track of how you feel and how well you are able to do your usual activities.

Answer every question by marking the answer as indicated. If you are unsure about how to answer a question, please give the best answer you can.

1. In general, would you say your health is:

(circle one)

Excellent	.1
Very good	.2
Good	.3
Fair	.4
Poor	.5

2. Compared to one year ago, how would you rate your health in general now?

(circle one)

Much better now than one year ago	.1
Somewhat better now than one year ago	.2
About the same as one year ago	.3
Somewhat worse now than one year ago	.4
Much worse now than one year ago	.5

3. The following items are about activities you might do during a typical day. Does
   your health now limit you in these activities? If so, how much?

(circle one number on each line)

ACTIVITIES	Yes, limited a lot	Yes, limited a little	No, not limited at all
a. **Vigorous activities**, such as running, lifting heavy objects, participating in strenuous sports	1	2	3
b. **Moderate activities**, such as moving a table, pushing a vacuum cleaner, bowling, or playing golf	1	2	3
c. Lifting or carrying groceries	1	2	3
d. Climbing **several** flights of stairs	1	2	3
e. Climbing **one** flight of stairs	1	2	3
f. Bending, kneeling, or stooping	1	2	3
g. Walking **more than a mile**	1	2	3
h. Walking **several blocks**	1	2	3
i. Walking **one block**	1	2	3
j. Bathing or dressing yourself	1	2	3

4. During the past 4 weeks, have you had any of the following problems with your
   work or other regular daily activities as a result of your physical health?

(circle one number on each line)

	Yes	No
a. Cut down on the **amount of time** you spent on work or other activities	1	2
b. **Accomplished less** than you would like	1	2
c. Were limited in the **kind** of work or other activities	1	2
d. Had **difficulty** performing the work or other activities (for example, it took extra effort)	1	2

5. During the <u>past 4 weeks</u>, have you had any of the following problems with your work or other regular daily activities <u>as a result of any emotional problems</u> (such as feeling depressed or anxious)?

(circle one number on each line)

	Yes	No
a. Cut down the **amount of time** you spent on work or other activities	1	2
b. **Accomplished less** than you would like	1	2
c. Didn't do work or other activities as **carefully** as usual	1	2

6. During the <u>past 4 weeks</u>, to what extent has your physical health or emotional problems interfered with your normal social activities with family, friends, neighbors, or groups?

(circle one)

Not at all 1

Slightly 2

Moderately 3

Quite a bit 4

Extremely 5

7. How much bodily pain have you had during the <u>past 4 weeks</u>?

None 1

Very mild 2

Mild 3

Moderate 4

Severe 5

Very severe 6

8. During the <u>past 4 weeks</u>, how much did <u>pain</u> interfere with your normal work (including both work outside the home and housework)?

                                                        (circle one)

        Not at all 1

        A little bit 2

        Moderately 3

        Quite a bit 4

        Extremely 5

9. These questions are about how you feel and how things have been with you <u>during the past 4 weeks</u>. For each question, please give the one answer that comes closest to the way you have been feeling. How much of the time <u>during the past 4 weeks</u> –

                                                       (circle on number on each line)

	All of the time	Most of the time	A good bit of the time	Some of the time	A little of the time	None of the time
a. Did you feel full of pep?	1	2	3	4	5	6
b. Have you been a very nervous person?	1	2	3	4	5	6
c. Have you felt so down in the dumps that nothing could cheer you up?	1	2	3	4	5	6
d. Have you felt calm and peaceful?	1	2	3	4	5	6
e. Did you have a lot of energy?	1	2	3	4	5	6
f. Have you felt downhearted and blue?	1	2	3	4	5	6
g. Did you feel worn out?	1	2	3	4	5	6
h. Have you been a happy person?	1	2	3	4	5	6
i. Did you feel tired?	1	2	3	4	5	6

10. During the <u>past 4 weeks</u>, how much of the time has your <u>physical health or emotional problems</u> interfered with your social activities (like visiting with friends, relatives, etc)?

(circle one)

All of the time 1

Most of the time 2

Some of the time 3

A little of the time 4

None of the time 5

11. How TRUE or FALSE is <u>each</u> of the following statements for you?

(circle one number on each line)

	Definately true	Mostly true	Don't know	Mostly false	Definitely false
a. I seem to get sick a little easier than other people	1	2	3	4	5
b. I am as healthy as anybody I know	1	2	3	4	5
c. I expect my health to get worse	1	2	3	4	5
d. My health is excellent	1	2	3	4	5

PATIENT HEALTH QUESTIONNAIRE (PHQ-9)

NAME: _____   DATE: _____

Over the *last 2 weeks,* how often have you been bothered by any of the following problems?
(use "✓" to indicate your answer)

	Not at all	Several days	More than half the days	Nearly every day
1. Little interest or pleasure in doing things	0	1	2	3
2. Feeling down, depressed, or hopeless	0	1	2	3
3. Trouble falling or staying asleep, or sleeping too much	0	1	2	3
4. Feeling tired or having little energy	0	1	2	3
5. Poor appetite or overeating	0	1	2	3
6. Feeling bad about yourself—or that you are a failure or have let yourself or your family down	0	1	2	3
7. Trouble concentrating on things, such as reading the newspaper or watching television	0	1	2	3
8. Moving or speaking so slowly that other people could have noticed. Or the opposite—being so fidgety or restless that you have been moving around a lot more than usual	0	1	2	3
9. Thoughts that you would be better off dead, or of hurting yourself in some way	0	1	2	3

add columns: _____ + _____ + _____

(Healthcare professional: For interpretation of TOTAL, please refer to accompanying scoring card.)   **TOTAL:** _____

10. If you checked off *any* problems, how *difficult* have these problems made it for you to do your work, take care of things at home, or get along with other people?	**Not difficult at all** _____ **Somewhat difficult** _____ **Very difficult** _____ **Extremely difficult** _____

PHQ-9 is adapted from PRIME MD TODAY, developed by Drs Robert L. Spitzer, Janet B.W. Williams, Kurt Kroenke, and colleagues, with an educational grant from Pfizer Inc. For research information, contact Dr Spitzer at rls8@columbia.edu. Use of the PHQ-9 may only be made in accordance with the Terms of Use available at *http://www.pfizer.com.* Copyright ©1999 Pfizer Inc. All rights reserved. PRIME MD TODAY is a trademark of Pfizer Inc.

ZT274388

Fold back this page before administering this questionnaire

PHQ-9 QUICK DEPRESSION ASSESSMENT

For initial diagnosis:

1. Patient completes PHQ-9 Quick Depression Assessment on accompanying tear-off pad.

2. If there are at least 4 ✓s in the blue highlighted section (including Questions #1 and #2), consider a depressive disorder. Add score to determine severity.

3. *Consider Major Depressive Disorder*
   —if there are at least 5 ✓s in the blue highlighted section (one of which corresponds to Question #1 or #2)

   Consider Other Depressive Disorder
   —if there are 2 to 4 ✓s in the blue highlighted section (one of which corresponds to Question #1 or #2)

Note: Since the questionnaire relies on patient self-report, all responses should be verified by the clinician and a definitive diagnosis made on clinical grounds, taking into account how well the patient understood the questionnaire, as well as other relevant information from the patient. Diagnoses of Major Depressive Disorder or Other Depressive Disorder also require impairment of social, occupational, or other important areas of functioning (Question #10) and ruling out normal bereavement, a history of a Manic Episode (Bipolar Disorder), and a physical disorder, medication, or other drug as the biological cause of the depressive symptoms.

To monitor severity over time for newly diagnosed patients or patients in current treatment for depression:

1. Patients may complete questionnaires at baseline and at regular intervals (eg, every 2 weeks) at home and bring them in at their next appointment for scoring or they may complete the questionnaire during each scheduled appointment.

2. Add up ✓s by column. For every ✓: Several days = 1   More than half the days = 2   Nearly every day = 3

3. Add together column scores to get a TOTAL score.

4. Refer to the accompanying PHQ-9 Scoring Card to interpret the TOTAL score.

5. Results may be included in patients' files to assist you in setting up a treatment goal, determining degree of response, as well as guiding treatment intervention.

Scoring—add up all checked boxes on PHQ-9

For every ✓: Not at all = 0; Several days = 1; More than half the days = 2; Nearly every day = 3

Interpretation of Total Score

Total Score	Depression Severity
0-4	None
5-9	Mild depression
10-14	Moderate depression
15-19	Moderately severe depression
20-27	Severe depression

The Medical Outcomes Study (MOS) Visit-Specific Questionnaire (VSQ)

Source: Rubin HR, et al: Patients ratings of outpatient visits in different practice settings. *JAMA* 270(7): 835-840, 1993.
Used with permission

Here are some questions about the visit you just made. In terms of your satisfaction, how would you rate each of the following?

(Check *One* Box on *Each* Line)

	Excellent 1	Very Good 2	Good 3	Fair 4	Poor 5
a. How *long* you waited to get an appointment	☐	☐	☐	☐	☐
b. Convenience of the *location* of the office	☐	☐	☐	☐	☐
c. Getting through to the office by *phone*	☐	☐	☐	☐	☐
d. Length of time *waiting* at the office	☐	☐	☐	☐	☐
e. Time spent *with the person* you saw	☐	☐	☐	☐	☐
f. *Explanation* of what was done for you	☐	☐	☐	☐	☐
g. The *technical skills* (thoroughness, carefulness, competence) of the person you saw	☐	☐	☐	☐	☐
h. The *personal manner* (courtesy, respect, sensitivity, friendliness) of the person you saw	☐	☐	☐	☐	☐
i. The visit *overall*	☐	☐	☐	☐	☐

Hospital Corporation of America Short-Form Patient Questionnaire

Source: Response Technologies, Hospital Corporation of America, © 1993. Used with permission from Columbia/HCA (Nashville, Tenn).

Hospital Quality: The Patient's Viewpoint

Please rate your hospital stay in each of the areas listed below in terms of whether it was excellent, very good, good, fair or poor. Please mark only one answer for each statement. (Check One Box on Each Line)

	Excellent	Very Good	Good	Fair	Poor	Does Not Apply
Admission: Entering the Hospital						
1. EFFICIENCY OF THE ADMITTING PROCEDURE: Ease of getting admitted, including the amount of time it took	☐	☐	☐	☐	☐	☐
2. ATTENTION OF ADMITTING STAFF TO YOUR INDIVIDUAL NEEDS: Their handling of your personal needs and wants	☐	☐	☐	☐	☐	☐
Your Daily Care in the Hospital						
3. SENSITIVITY TO PROBLEMS: Sensitivity of hospital staff to your special problems or concerns	☐	☐	☐	☐	☐	☐
4. COORDINATION OF CARE: The teamwork of all the hospital staff who took care of you	☐	☐	☐	☐	☐	☐
Keeping You Informed						
5. EASE OF GETTING INFORMATION: Willingness of hospital staff to answer your questions	☐	☐	☐	☐	☐	☐
6. INSTRUCTIONS: How well nurses and other staff explained about tests, treatments and what to expect	☐	☐	☐	☐	☐	☐
7. INFORMING FAMILY OR FRIENDS: How well they were kept informed about your condition and needs	☐	☐	☐	☐	☐	☐
Your Nurses						
8. SKILL OF NURSES: How well things were done, like giving medicine and handling IVs	☐	☐	☐	☐	☐	☐
9. ATTENTION OF NURSES TO YOUR CONDITION: How often nurses checked on you to keep track of how you were doing	☐	☐	☐	☐	☐	☐
10. NURSING STAFF RESPONSE TO YOUR CALLS: How quick they were to help	☐	☐	☐	☐	☐	☐
11. CONCERN AND CARING BY NURSES: Courtesy and respect you were given; friendliness and kindness	☐	☐	☐	☐	☐	☐
Your Doctor						
12. ATTENTION OF DOCTOR TO YOUR CONDITION: How often doctors checked on you to keep track of how you were doing	☐	☐	☐	☐	☐	☐
13. CONCERN AND CARING BY DOCTORS: Courtesy and respect you were given; friendliness and kindness	☐	☐	☐	☐	☐	☐
14. SKILL OF DOCTORS: Ability to diagnose problems, thoroughness of examination, and skill in treating your condition	☐	☐	☐	☐	☐	☐
15. INFORMATION GIVEN BY DOCTORS: Information given about your illness and treatment; what to do after leaving the hospital	☐	☐	☐	☐	☐	☐
Other Hospital Staff						
16. HOUSEKEEPING STAFF: How well they did their jobs and how they acted towards you	☐	☐	☐	☐	☐	☐
17. LABORATORY STAFF: How well they did their jobs and how they acted towards you	☐	☐	☐	☐	☐	☐
18. IV STARTERS: Skill of staff who started your IV	☐	☐	☐	☐	☐	☐

(continued on next page)

	Excellent	Very Good	Good	Fair	Poor	Does Not Apply
Living Arrangements						
19. RESTFULNESS OF ATMOSPHERE: Amount of peace and quiet	☐	☐	☐	☐	☐	☐
20. HOSPITAL BUILDING: How would you rate the hospital building overall	☐	☐	☐	☐	☐	☐
Discharge: Leaving the Hospital						
21. DISCHARGE PROCEDURES: Time it took to be discharged from the hospital and how efficiently it was handled	☐	☐	☐	☐	☐	☐
22. DISCHARGE INSTRUCTIONS: How clearly and completely you were told what to do and what to expect when you left the hospital	☐	☐	☐	☐	☐	☐
Billing by Hospital						
23. EXPLANATIONS ABOUT YOUR HOSPITAL BILLS: The accuracy of information and willingness to answer your questions about finances	☐	☐	☐	☐	☐	☐
24. EFFICIENCY OF BILLING: How fast you got your bill, how accurate and understandable it was	☐	☐	☐	☐	☐	☐

Facts About You (FOR STATISTICAL PURPOSES ONLY)

25. Are you (the patient) male or female? ☐ Male ☐ Female

26. Where did you stay in the hospital?
In a section of the hospital for. . . (mark all that apply)

☐ Adult Medical ☐ Children/Maternity
☐ Critical Care ☐ Rehabilitation
☐ Heart/Coronary Care ☐ Mental Health
☐ Other – Please specify _____

27. In what year were you (the patient) born? _____

28. On what date were you (will you be) discharged from the hospital?
Example: January 1, 1991. _____

Looking Back on Your Care	Excellent	Very Good	Good	Fair	Poor	Does Not Apply
29. THE OUTCOME OF YOUR HOSPITAL STAY: How much you were helped by the hospitalization	☐	☐	☐	☐	☐	☐

30. Would you return to this hospital if you needed to be hospitalized again?

☐ Definitely Yes ☐ Definitely Not
☐ Probably Yes ☐ Does Not Apply (ie, because do
☐ Probably Not   not live near hospital)

Why or why not? _____

31. Did anything very good happen during your stay in the hospital that you did not expect? If so, please tell us what it was.

_____

32. Did anything bad happen during your stay in the hospital that you did not expect? If so, please tell us what it was.

_____

33. We may wish to call you to learn more about your hospital stay. If you would like to give us permission to contact you, please write your name and phone number in the space provided.

Name _____ Phone _____

CAHPS® Hospital Survey

SURVEY INSTRUCTIONS

◆ You should only fill out this survey if you were the patient during the hospital stay named in the cover letter. Do not fill out this survey if you were not the patient.

◆ Answer <u>all</u> the questions by checking the box to the left of your answer.

◆ You are sometimes told to skip over some questions in this survey. When this happens you will see an arrow with a note that tells you what question to answer next, like this:

      ☐   Yes
      ☑   No   ➜ *If No, Go to Question 1 on Page 1*

You may notice a number on the cover of this survey. This number is ONLY used to let us know if you returned your survey so we don't have to send you reminders.
Please note: Questions 1-22 in this survey are part of a national initiative to measure the quality   of care in hospitals.

Please answer the questions in this survey about your stay at the hospital named on the cover. Do not include any other hospital stay in your answers.

YOUR CARE FROM NURSES

1.   **During this hospital stay, how often did nurses treat you with <u>courtesy and respect</u>?**

      ¹☐ Never
      ²☐ Sometimes
      ³☐ Usually
      ⁴☐ Always

2. During this hospital stay, how often did nurses <u>listen carefully to you</u>?

¹☐ Never
²☐ Sometimes
³☐ Usually
⁴☐ Always

3. During this hospital stay, how often did nurses <u>explain things</u> in a way you could understand?

¹☐ Never
²☐ Sometimes
³☐ Usually
⁴☐ Always

4. During this hospital stay, after you pressed the call button, how often did you get help as soon as you wanted it?

¹☐ Never
²☐ Sometimes
³☐ Usually
⁴☐ Always
⁹☐ I never pressed the call button

YOUR CARE FROM DOCTORS

5. During this hospital stay, how often did doctors treat you with <u>courtesy and respect</u>?

¹☐ Never
²☐ Sometimes
³☐ Usually
⁴☐ Always

6. During this hospital stay, how often did doctors <u>listen carefully to you</u>?

¹☐ Never
²☐ Sometimes

3☐ Usually

4☐ Always

7. **During this hospital stay, how often did doctors <u>explain things</u> in a way you could understand?**

1☐ Never

2☐ Sometimes

3☐ Usually

4☐ Always

THE HOSPITAL ENVIRONMENT

8. **During this hospital stay, how often were your room and bathroom kept clean?**

1☐ Never

2☐ Sometimes

3☐ Usually

4☐ Always

9. **During this hospital stay, how often was the area around your room quiet at night?**

1☐ Never

2☐ Sometimes

3☐ Usually

4☐ Always

YOUR EXPERIENCES IN THIS HOSPITAL

10. **During this hospital stay, did you need help from nurses or other hospital staff in getting to the bathroom or in using a bedpan?**

1☐ Yes

2☐ No ➔ **If No, Go to Question 12**

11. **How often did you get help in getting to the bathroom or in using a bedpan as soon as you wanted?**

1☐ Never

2☐ Sometimes

3☐ Usually

[4] □ Always

12. During this hospital stay, did you need medicine for pain?

[1] □ Yes
[2] □ No ➜ **If No, Go to Question 15**

13. During this hospital stay, how often was your pain well controlled?

[1] □ Never
[2] □ Sometimes
[3] □ Usually
[4] □ Always

14. During this hospital stay, how often did the hospital staff do everything they could to help you with your pain?

[1] □ Never
[2] □ Sometimes
[3] □ Usually
[4] □ Always

15. During this hospital stay, were you given any medicine that you had not taken before?

[1] □ Yes
[2] □ No ➜ **If No, Go to Question 18**

16. Before giving you any new medicine, how often did hospital staff tell you what the medicine was for?

[1] □ Never
[2] □ Sometimes
[3] □ Usually
[4] □ Always

17. Before giving you any new medicine, how often did hospital staff describe possible side effects in a way you could understand?

[1] □ Never

²☐ Sometimes
³☐ Usually
⁴☐ Always

WHEN YOU LEFT THE HOSPITAL

18. After you left the hospital, did you go directly to your own home, to someone else's home, or to another health facility?

¹☐ Own home
²☐ Someone else's home
³☐ Another health facility ➔   If Another, Go to Question 21

19. During this hospital stay, did doctors, nurses or other hospital staff talk with you about whether you would have the help you needed when you left the hospital?

¹☐ Yes
²☐ No

20. During this hospital stay, did you get information in writing about what symptoms or health problems to look out for after you left the hospital?

¹☐ Yes
²☐ No

OVERALL RATING OF HOSPITAL

Please answer the following questions about your stay at the hospital named on the cover. Do not include any other hospital stays in your answer.

21. Using any number from 0 to 10, where 0 is the worst hospital possible and 10 is the best hospital possible, what number would you use to rate this hospital during your stay?

⁰☐ 0   Worst hospital possible
¹☐ 1
²☐ 2
³☐ 3
⁴☐ 4
⁵☐ 5
⁶☐ 6

⁷☐　7

⁸☐　8

⁹☐　9

¹⁰☐　10　　　Best hospital possible

22.　Would you recommend this hospital to your friends and family?

¹☐ Definitely no

²☐ Probably no

³☐ Probably yes

⁴☐ Definitely yes

ABOUT YOU

There are only a few remaining items left.

23.　In general, how would you rate your overall health?

¹☐ Excellent

²☐ Very good

³☐ Good

⁴☐ Fair

⁵☐ Poor

24.　What is the highest grade or level of school that you have <u>completed</u>?

¹☐ 8th grade or less

²☐ Some high school, but did not graduate

³☐ High school graduate or GED

⁴☐ Some college or 2-year degree

⁵☐ 4-year college graduate

⁶☐ More than 4-year college degree

25.　Are you of Spanish, Hispanic or Latino origin or descent?

¹☐ No, not Spanish/Hispanic/Latino

²☐ Yes, Puerto Rican

³☐ Yes, Mexican, Mexican American, Chicano

⁴☐ Yes, Cuban

[5]☐ Yes, other Spanish/Hispanic/Latino

26. What is your race? Please choose one or more.

[1]☐ White
[2]☐ Black or African American
[3]☐ Asian
[4]☐ Native Hawaiian or other Pacific Islander
[5]☐ American Indian or Alaska Native

27. What language do you <u>mainly</u> speak at home?

[1]☐ English
[2]☐ Spanish
[8]☐ Some other language (please print): _____

THANK YOU

Please return the completed survey in the postage-paid envelope.

CAHPS® Clinician & Group Survey

Adult Primary Care Questionnaire

October 2006

All information that would let someone identify you or your family will be kept private. {VENDOR NAME} will not share your personal information with anyone without your OK. You may choose to answer this survey or not. If you choose not to, this will not affect the benefits you get.

*Your responses to this survey are completely **confidential**. Once you complete the survey, place it in the envelope that was provided, seal the envelope, and return the envelope to [INSERT VENDOR ADDRESS].*

*You may notice a number on the cover of this survey. This number is **only** used to let us know if you returned your survey so we don't have to send you reminders.*

If you want to know more about this study, please call XXX-XXX-XXXX.

About the Never/Always Response Scale

This survey employs the standard CAHPS four-point response scale of "Never/Sometimes/Usually/Always." Several early adopters have fielded the survey using an alternative six-point response scale: "Never/Almost Never/Sometimes/Usually/Almost Always/Always." The CAHPS Consortium recommends that early adopters continue to use the six-point response scale and will continue to examine the performance of the four-point and six-point response scales in the context of this survey.

CAHPS Clinician & Group Survey – Adult Questionnaire

Core Items

YOUR DOCTOR

1. **Our records show that you got care from the doctor named below in the last 12 months.**

    NAME OF DOCTOR LABEL GOES HERE

    Is that right?

    ¹ ☐ Yes➔ **If Yes, Go to Question 2**
    ² ☐ No➔ **If No, Go to Question 26**

The questions in this survey booklet will refer to the doctor named in Question 1 as "this doctor." Please think of that doctor as you answer the survey.

2. **Is this the doctor you usually see if you need a check-up, want advice about a health problem, or get sick or hurt?**

    ¹ ☐ Yes
    ² ☐ No

3. **How long have you been going to this doctor?**

    ¹ ☐ Less than 6 months
    ² ☐ At least 6 months but less than 1 year
    ³ ☐ At least 1 year but less than 3 years
    ⁴ ☐ At least 3 years but less than 5 years
    ⁵ ☐ 5 years or more

YOUR CARE FROM THIS DOCTOR IN THE LAST 12 MONTHS

These questions ask about <u>your own</u> health care. Do <u>not</u> include care you got when you stayed overnight in a hospital. Do <u>not</u> include the times you went for dental care visits.

4.   In the last 12 months, how many times did you visit this doctor to get care for yourself?

   ^{1}☐ None ➜ **If None, Go to Question 26**
   ^{2}☐ 1
   ^{3}☐ 2
   ^{4}☐ 3
   ^{5}☐ 4
   ^{6}☐ 5 to 9
   ^{7}☐ 10 or more

5.   In the last 12 months, did you phone this doctor's office to get an appointment for an illness, injury or condition that <u>needed care right away</u>?

   ^{1}☐ Yes

   ^{2}☐ No ➜ **If No, Go to Question 7**

6.   In the last 12 months, when you phoned this doctor's office to get an appointment for <u>care you needed right away</u>, how often did you get an appointment as soon as you thought you needed it?

   ^{1}☐ Never
   ^{2}☐ Sometimes
   ^{3}☐ Usually
   ^{4}☐ Always

7.   In the last 12 months, did you make any appointments for a <u>check-up or routine care</u> with this doctor?

   ^{1}☐ Yes

   ^{2}☐ No ➜ **If No, Go to Question 9**

8.   In the last 12 months, when you made an appointment for a <u>check-up or routine care</u> with this doctor, how often did you get an appointment as soon as you thought you needed it?

   ¹☐ Never

   ²☐ Sometimes

   ³☐ Usually

   ⁴☐ Always

9.   In the last 12 months, did you phone this doctor's office with a medical question <u>during</u> regular office hours?

   ¹☐ Yes

   ²☐ No➔ If No, Go to Question 11

10.   In the last 12 months, when you phoned this doctor's office during regular office hours, how often did you get an answer to your medical question that same day?

   ¹☐ Never

   ²☐ Sometimes

   ³☐ Usually

   ⁴☐ Always

11.   In the last 12 months, did you phone this doctor's office with a medical question <u>after</u> regular office hours?

   ¹☐ Yes

   ²☐ No➔ If No, Go to Question 13

12.   In the last 12 months, when you phoned this doctor's office after regular office hours, how often did you get an answer to your medical question as soon as you needed?

   ¹☐ Never

   ²☐ Sometimes

   ³☐ Usually

   ⁴☐ Always

13. **Wait time includes time spent in the waiting room and exam room. In the last 12 months, how often did you see this doctor <u>within 15 minutes</u> of your appointment time?**

    [1] ☐ Never
    [2] ☐ Sometimes
    [3] ☐ Usually
    [4] ☐ Always

14. **In the last 12 months, how often did this doctor explain things in a way that was easy to understand?**

    [1] ☐ Never
    [2] ☐ Sometimes
    [3] ☐ Usually
    [4] ☐ Always

15. **In the last 12 months, how often did this doctor listen carefully to you?**

    [1] ☐ Never
    [2] ☐ Sometimes
    [3] ☐ Usually
    [4] ☐ Always

16. **In the last 12 months, did you talk with this doctor about any health problems or concerns?**

    [1] ☐ Yes
    [2] ☐ No → **If No, Go to Question 18**

17. **In the last 12 months, how often did this doctor give you easy to understand instructions about taking care of these health problems or concerns?**

    [1] ☐ Never
    [2] ☐ Sometimes
    [3] ☐ Usually
    [4] ☐ Always

18.   In the last 12 months, how often did this doctor seem to know the important information about your medical history?

¹☐ Never
²☐ Sometimes
³☐ Usually
⁴☐ Always

19.   In the last 12 months, how often did this doctor show respect for what you had to say?

¹☐ Never
²☐ Sometimes
³☐ Usually
⁴☐ Always

20.   In the last 12 months, how often did this doctor spend enough time with you?

¹☐ Never
²☐ Sometimes
³☐ Usually
⁴☐ Always

21.   In the last 12 months, did this doctor order a blood test, x-ray or other test for you?

¹☐ Yes
²☐ No➔ If No, Go to Question 23

22.   In the last 12 months, when this doctor ordered a blood text, x-ray or other test for you, how often did someone from this doctor's office follow up to give you those results?

¹☐ Never
²☐ Sometimes
³☐ Usually
⁴☐ Always

23. **Using any number from 0 to 10, where 0 is the worst doctor possible and 10 is the best doctor possible, what number would you use to rate this doctor?**

☐ 0 Worst doctor possible

☐ 1

☐ 2

☐ 3

☐ 4

☐ 5

☐ 6

☐ 7

☐ 8

☐ 9

☐ 10 Best doctor possible

CLERKS AND RECEPTIONISTS AT THIS DOCTOR'S OFFICE

24. **In the last 12 months, how often were clerks and receptionists at this doctor's office as helpful as you thought they should be?**

[1] ☐ Never

[2] ☐ Sometimes

[3] ☐ Usually

[4] ☐ Always

25. **In the last 12 months, how often did clerks and receptionists at this doctor's office treat you with courtesy and respect?**

[1] ☐ Never

[2] ☐ Sometimes

[3] ☐ Usually

[4] ☐ Always

ABOUT YOU

26. **In general, how would you rate your overall health?**

    [1]☐ Excellent
    [2]☐ Very good
    [3]☐ Good
    [4]☐ Fair
    [5]☐ Poor

27. **In the past 12 months, have you seen a doctor or other health provider 3 or more times for the same condition or problem?**

    [1]☐ Yes
    [2]☐ No➔ **If No, Go to Question 29**

28. **Is this a condition or problem that has lasted for at least 3 months? Do <u>not</u> include pregnancy or menopause.**

    [1]☐ Yes
    [2]☐ No

29 **Do you now need or take medicine prescribed by a doctor? Do <u>not</u> include birth control.**

    ☐ Yes
    ☐ No➔ **If No, Go to Question 31**

30. **Is this medicine to treat a condition that has lasted for at least 3 months? Do <u>not</u> include pregnancy or menopause.**

    [1]☐ Yes
    [2]☐ No

31. **What is your age?**

    [1]☐ 18 to 24
    [2]☐ 25 to 34
    [3]☐ 35 to 44
    [4]☐ 45 to 54
    [5]☐ 55 to 64
    [6]☐ 65 to 74
    [7]☐ 75 or older

32.   Are you male or female?

[1] ☐ Male
[2] ☐ Female

33.   What is the highest grade or level of school that you have completed?

[1] ☐ 8th grade or less
[2] ☐ Some high school, but did not graduate
[3] ☐ High school graduate or GED
[4] ☐ Some college or 2-year degree
[5] ☐ 4-year college graduate
[6] ☐ More than 4-year college degree

34.   Are you of Hispanic or Latino origin or descent?

[1] ☐ Yes, Hispanic or Latino
[2] ☐ No, not Hispanic or Latino

35.   What is your race? Please mark one or more.

[1] ☐ White
[2] ☐ Black or African American
[3] ☐ Asian
[4] ☐ Native Hawaiian or Other Pacific Islander
[5] ☐ American Indian or Alaskan Native
[6] ☐ Other

THANK YOU

Please return the completed survey in the postage-paid envelope.

CAHPS® Clinician & Group Survey- Adult Primary Care Questionnaire. Agency for Healthcare Research and Quality, Rockville, MD. December 2006.
https://www.cahps.ahrq.gov/content/products/CG/PROD_CG_Adult_Primary.htm

Return to the CAHPS Clinician & Group Survey Page
CAHPS Home Page

Patient Utilization Questions

Source: Items 1–3: Eugene C. Nelson, Dartmouth Medical School, 1997. Adapted from the Medical Outcomes Study, The RAND Corporation, 1986. Used with permission. Items 4–9: CA HPS® Clinician and Group Survey Adult Primary Care Questionnaire. AHRQ 2006. pp. 24–26.

Cost of Care: Hospitals and Clinical Visits

1. In the last 12 months, how many times have you been a patient in a <u>hospital</u> overnight or longer?

    0   1   2   3   or more times

2. In the last 6 months, how many times did you see a <u>medical doctor</u>? (Do not count times while an overnight patient in a hospital.)

    0   1   2   3   4   5   6 or more times

3. In the last 6 months, how many times did you see a <u>mental health specialist</u> for a personal or emotional problem?

    0   1   2   3   4   5   6 or more times

Cost of Care: (Prescriptions)

4. In the last 12 months, did you take any <u>prescription medicine</u>?

    Yes   No

5. In the last 12 months, were you ever worried or <u>concerned about the cost</u> of your prescription medicine?

    Yes   No

6. In the last 12 months, did you and your doctor <u>talk about the cost</u> of your prescription medicine?

    Yes   No

Cost of Care: (Tests)

7. In the last 12 months, did a doctor order a <u>blood test, x-ray or other test</u> for you?

    Yes   No

8. In the last 12 months, were you ever worried or <u>concerned about the cost</u> of your blood tests, x-rays or other tests?

    Yes   No

9. In the last 12 months, did you and your doctor <u>talk about the cost</u> of your blood tests, x-rays or other tests?

Yes   No

Appendix D

COLLECTING DATA: PRINCIPLES AND GUIDELINES FOR SUCCESS

Eugene C. Nelson

Background

Curiosity, observation, reflection, experimentation, and measurement are some of the fundamental skills that support self-generated improvement in clinical practice. Elsewhere in this book we have explored observation, reflection, and experimentation using the scientific method and Plan-Do-Study-Act (PDSA) and Standardize-Do-Study-Act (SDSA) framework. This appendix offers brief guidance on how to design measurement processes into daily clinical work to promote practice-based learning and improvement.

A substantial body of literature describes practice-based measurement in greater detail. Readers can refer to the following resources in particular:

- Nelson E.C., et al.: Data and measurement in clinical microsystems: Part 2. Creating a rich information environment. *Jt Comm J Qual Saf* 29:5-15, Jan. 2003.
- Weinstein J., et al.: Designing an ambulatory clinical practice for outcomes improvement: From vision to reality: The Spine Center at Dartmouth-Hitchcock, year one. *Qual Manag Health Care* 8:1–20, Winter 2000.
- Hess A.M., et al.: Building an idealized measurement system to improve clinical office practice performance. *Manag Care Q* 7:22–34, Summer 1999.
- Nelson E.C., et al.: Building measurement and data collection into medical practice. *Ann Intern Med* 128:460–466, Mar. 15, 1998.
- Nelson E.C., et al.: Report cards or instrument panels: Who needs what? *Jt Comm J Qual Improv* 21:155–166, Apr. 1995.

In addition, because building measurement into busy clinical practice requires a deep understanding of how things work today and how things could work in the future, we include tips on using flowcharts and process maps to track flow of data and information. For more on process mapping and flowcharting, please also refer to the following works:

- George M.L., et al.: *The Lean Six Sigma Pocket Toolbook.* New York City: McGraw-Hill, 2005.
- Scholtes P.R., Joiner B.L., Streibel B.J.: *The Team Handbook,* 3rd ed. Madison, WI: Oriel, Inc., 2003.
- Rother M., Shook J.: *Learning to See: Value Stream Mapping to Add Value and Eliminate Muda.* Brookline, MA: The Lean Enterprise Institute, 1998.

Principles for Using Data in Clinical Practice for Learning and Improvement[1]

1. Keep Measurement Simple. Think Big and Start Small

Always see the solution (or the end result or the outcome) as a matter of causes and effects that interact dynamically over time (that is, a web of causation).[1] To begin, contemplate the web in its entirety, but start by measuring only a few key, high-leverage causal elements (process and case mix variables) and one or two critical outcomes. As time passes, data on more of the system variables (inputs, processes, outputs, feedback loops) can be captured for learning, reflection, and taking action.

2. More Data Are Not Necessarily Better Data. Seek Usefulness, Not Perfection, in Measures

Be clear about what question must be answered and then target data collection to find the answer. More data are not necessarily better data. Collecting too much data incurs many risks: The work of collection might preclude cooperation from those who have to do it, more data might yield more collection and recording errors, data collection can be expensive, and finally, the importance of the effort might be compromised if those for whom it is to provide help regard these measures as irrelevant. Discontinue measures when it is determined that new measures are more useful.

3. Write Down the Operational Definitions of Measures

The quality of measurement values is contingent on the accuracy of the individual data elements. Having and following clear operational definitions is essential for recording data and creating measures if the data are to be reliable and valid. In addition, interpreting data is easier when documented definitions are readily available. When using a newly created data collection form, make full use of self-coding data sheets that reflect the operational definition in the layout of the question and the response choices, and that have operational definitions printed on the front or back side of the data collection form.

4. Use a Balanced Set of Input, Process, Outcome, and Cost Measures

To gain insight, it is necessary to deepen one's understanding of the web of causation. This involves capturing sources of causation (inputs), intervening events (processes), and transitions in important results (outcomes and costs) of the system that is to be managed and improved. Instrument panels provide critical, real-time information on the system's total performance and can prompt the user to make wise decisions and, if necessary, make rapid midcourse corrections.[2] The use of inclusive frameworks (such as structure-process-outcome, value compass thinking, and microsystem approaches) can help to reveal which parts of the system are important for measurement and which interactions between parts are most variable and critical.

5. Build Measurement into Daily Work and Job Descriptions

Data collection, analysis, and display should be designed into the flow of medical practice. Measurement is already built into some clinical practice routines, for example, taking vital signs at the beginning of an office visit or cardiac monitoring of patients in coronary care units. New measurements can be designed into clinical care routines and into the job descriptions of people who are involved in the care of patients. The key idea is to capture the right data, correctly, and to use them immediately and repeatedly.

6. Use Qualitative and Quantitative Data

Quantitative data can provide limited and precise slices of how the system is performing and how the patient is doing. Maps of causes and effects and of feedback loops can also provide a sense of how different measures interrelate. Quantitative data provide a simplified model of real-ity. Qualitative data (observations, critical incidents, verbatim comments, unsolicited compliments and complaints) can provide a richer understanding of the underlying background from which the quantitative data emerge.

7. Use Available Data if Possible; Otherwise, Measure Small Representative Samples

All systems are constantly throwing off data that can be used for learning, managing, researching, and taking action. Sometimes the data produced by the system are already being "caught" with sufficient accuracy: What needs to be done is to retrieve, analyze, and display the data in a useful manner. If the data exist and are sufficiently accurate, use them. Many times, however, the question that is posed cannot be answered by reprocessing "caught" data. Under these conditions, new data must be gathered prospectively. In this case, begin by gathering data on small, representative, time-ordered samples. Using a systematic or random sample—or selecting a judgment sample—to reflect how the system is performing under different known conditions can be helpful.

8. Display Key Measures (for Viewing by Staff and Patients) That Demonstrate Trends Over Time

Data are not self-actuating; they must be analyzed, displayed, and interpreted to create the conditions for taking intelligent action. Graphic visual displays of data can help people to interpret results and to create the conditions for taking such action. Consider building viewable "data walls" or "storyboards" to create a physical, visual environment through which data can be communicated in a timely manner. One of the most powerful ways for displaying data is to use statistical process control methods. Graphically tracking results—or drivers of results—can help us gain insight to inform appropriate action on the basis of historical trends, current values, and thus probable future outcomes.

9. Develop a Measurement Team and Establish Ownership

Sharing the burden of measurement lightens the load for everyone. Understanding and participation can be broadened by inviting key people, with different professional skills and training, to take responsibility for different facets of data collection and analysis. In general, a small group of interested people is needed to create a data environment that will be most useful to members of the microsystem who work together to deliver medical care. This small measurement team can develop operational definitions and data management plans, which can be reviewed by the entire staff and by patients for consensus and implementation.

Guidelines for Designing a Measurement Process: A 12-Pack of Suggestions

Aim, Users, Uses

1. Ensure that intended use and analysis of data are clear.
2. Ensure that the methods of organizing, displaying, and summarizing data allow study of factors that might have important effects on the results.

Definitions

3. Develop clear definitions of how observations are to be translated into measurements or evaluations.
4. Ensure that the method of measurement results in obtaining the intended information.
5. Ensure that the measurement methods to be used are clear and simple and minimize on-the-spot decision making.

Planning

6. Design measurement that isn't too big–less is more.
7. Embed measurement and data collection into the daily activities of the system under study.
8. Ensure that measurement and data analysis are timely.
9. Develop a plan for training those who will make the measurements, record the data, and keep a diary for recording auxiliary information.
10. Perform pilot studies of definitions, methods of measurement, data collection forms, and training.
11. Determine who is responsible for the measurement process.

12. Inform all affected associates about the purpose of collecting data.

Process Mapping Tips

1. Start at a high level, and go "lower" until you find obvious things to change.
2. Align the boundaries with the aim.
3. Map the actual process.
4. Identify the steps as the patient would go through them.
5. Get general agreement from all the essential players.
6. Find the process constraints—"likely early leverage."
7. Develop the key supportive processes that contribute to the flow.
8. Benchmark meaningfully with knowledge of the "home" results and the process.
9. Keep track of the obvious things worth trying to change.

For more information on flowcharting please see:

- Scholtes P.R., Joiner B.L., Streibel B.J.: *The Team Handbook: How to Use Teams to Improve Quality,* 3rd ed. Madison, WI: Oriel, Inc., 2003.
- George M., et al.: *The Lean Six Sigma Pocket Tool Book.* New York City: McGraw Hill, 2005.
- Nelson E.C, Batalden P.B., Godfrey M.M.: *Quality by Design: A Clinical Microsystem Approach.* San Francisco: Jossey-Bass, 2007.

References
1. McMahon B., Pugh T.: *Epidemiology Principles and Methods.* New York City: Little, Brown and Company, 1970.
2. Nelson E.C., et al.: Report cards or instrument panels: Who needs what? *Jt Comm J Qual Improv* 21:155–166, Apr. 1995.
3. For a more detailed review of these principles, please see: Nelson E.C., et al.: Using data to improve medical practice by measuring processes and outcomes of care. *Jt Comm J Qual Improv* 26:667–685, Dec. 2000.

Appendix E

Surfing the Web: A Starter Set of Internet Sites for Practice-Based Learning and Health Care Improvement

Eugene C. Nelson

Purpose

The Internet is a dynamic and evolving resource for information, ideas, and useful tools that can facilitate practice-based learning and improvement. Specific Web sites might be very helpful to individuals who wish to do the following:

- Improve health care.
- Develop practice-based learning groups.
- Scan the literature for benchmarking data and evidence-based best practices.
- Identify clinical practice guidelines and quality metrics.
- Create survey instruments to assess local performance.
- Dig more deeply into sources of information and knowledge.

In this appendix, we provide a small starter set of Web sites that are useful for one or more of these purposes. This list is certainly not exhaustive but is representative of Web sites that the editors have found useful for initiation of improvement projects. The sites are listed alphabetically. More can be learned about what each site (as last accessed on June 5, 2007) has to offer by making a visit to the site and learning firsthand.

Accreditation Council for Graduate Medical Education (ACGME): *Home Page*
http://www.acgme.org/acWebsite/home/home.asp

Agency for Healthcare Research and Quality (AHRQ): *Home Page*
http://www.ahrq.gov/

American Hospital Association (AHA): *Quality and Patient Safety*
http://www.aha.org/aha_app/issues/Quality-and-Patient-Safety

American Medical Association (AMA): *Home Page*
http://www.ama-assn.org/

Baldrige National Quality Program: *Home Page*
http://www.quality.nist.gov/

British Medical Journal (BMJ): *Home Page*
http://www.bmj.com/

Clinical Microsystems: *Home Page*
http://www.clinicalmicrosystem.org/

Healthcare Improvement Skills Center: *Home Page*
http://www.improvementskills.org/

How's Your Health: *Home Page*
http://www.howsyourhealth.org/

Ideal Micropractices: *Home Page*
http://www.idealmicropractice.com/

Improvement Foundation: *Home Page*
http://www.improvementfoundation.org/View.aspx?page=/default.html

Institute for Clinical Systems Improvement (ICSI): *Home Page*
http://www.icsi.org/

Institute for Family-Centered Care: *Home Page*
http://www.familycenteredcare.org/

Institute for Healthcare Improvement (IHI): *Home Page*
http://www.ihi.org/ihi

Institute for Safe Medication Practices (ISMP): *Home Page*

http://www.ismp.org/

Institute of Medicine (IOM): *Home Page*

http://www.iom.edu/

Intermountain Healthcare (IHC): *Intermountain Clinical Programs*

http://intermountainhealthcare.org/xp/public/physician/clinicalprograms/

The Joint Commission: *Home Page*

http://www.jointcommission.org/

The Joint Commission International Center for Patient Safety (ICPS): *Home Page*

http://www.jcipatientsafety.org/

Joint Commission Resources: *Home Page*

http://www.jcrinc.com/

Journal of the American Medical Association (JAMA): *Home Page*

http://jama.ama-assn.org/

National Library of Medicine (NLM): *Home Page*

http://www.nlm.nih.gov/

National Patient Safety Foundation (NPSF): *Home Page*

http://www.npsf.org/

New England Journal of Medicine (NEJM): Home Page

http://content.nejm.org/

Veterans Administration National Center for Patient Safety (VA NCPS): *National Center for Patient Safety 2004 Falls Toolkit*

http://www.va.gov/ncps/SafetyTopics/fallstoolkit/index.html

GLOSSARY

ACGME The Accreditation Council for Graduate Medical Education (ACGME) is responsible for the accreditation of post-MD medical training programs within the United States. Accreditation is accomplished through a peer review process and is based on established standards and guidelines.

benchmark A measure of an outcome or a topic of interest that is usually expressed in the form of a number value. Sometimes referred to as the best-known value, but often used to refer to a target value that might represent an average value or a desired value.

benchmarking In general, the search for best practices that consistently produce best-in-the-world results. A systematic process of continuously measuring an organization's critical business processes and results against leaders anywhere in the world to gain information that will help the organization take action to improve its performance. Steps include planning the study, collecting information, analyzing results, and implementing improvements.

brainstorming The group process technique that generates creative ideas through an interactive process.

care process model A care process model (CPM) is an approach developed by Intermountain Healthcare to design best practices and evidence-based care into the routine flow of health care delivery in all related clinical microsystems in a large, integrated health system. A CPM includes the evidence base, clinical guidelines, decision support, patient and provider education materials, outcomes tracking, and periodic performance feedback to frontline clinical systems and to individual clinicians.

change concepts A family of change ideas that represent a general method for improving a process. The general method for improving a process can be adapted to work in a specific process. For example, the change concept of "turning the customer into the supplier" can be used to redesign or design many different, specific process flows.

clinical guideline (or pathway) A standard set of recommendations to guide care for patients with common health problems. Often takes the form of a checklist indicating what should be done at what point in time or at what stage of treatment.

clinical improvement The ongoing process of redesigning the delivery of clinical care, using the Plan-Do-Study-Act (PDSA) method, to improve value of care.

clinical microsystems, mesosystems, macrosystems Clinical microsystems are small systems, and they are the places where patients, families, and caregivers meet. Wherever a patient interacts with one or more caregivers to deal with a health matter there is, by definition, a clinical microsystem. Clinical microsystems are the front lines of care delivery and the naturally occurring building blocks of the health care delivery system. Common examples are a pediatric practice, an orthopedic practice, an emergency room, a medical emergency team, an intensive care unit, and a cardiac surgery team. Clinical mesosystems are midsize systems and are collections (or clusters) of microsystems that contribute to the care of the patient as he or she moves through the health care system over time. Examples are all the clinical units that contribute to the provision of obstetrical care, trauma care, cardiovascular care, cancer care, and mental health care. Clinical macrosystems are larger systems that include multiple microsystems and mesosystems. They usually have names such as "St. James Hospital" or "Gotham City Health System." Common examples are a hospital, a multispecialty group practice, a nursing home, or an integrated health system.

clinical protocol (or algorithm) Sharply focused instructions to provide specific recommendations on what to do for a discrete aspect of clinical care (for example, ventilator management, making a diagnosis, selecting a drug). Protocols, in contrast to guidelines, tend to be narrower in scope and more directive.

CMS The Centers for Medicare & Medicaid Services (CMS) is a U.S. federal governmental agency that manages Medicare and Medicaid and administers a wide array of programs and initiatives that aim to improve the quality, safety, and costs of care.

coach A person who supports clinical improvement effort with improvement experience, improvement knowledge, and organizational leadership.

consensus The decision-making process that explores and respects all team members' opinions and arrives at a decision that all team members can accept.

control chart A graphic format for displaying information that shows data points in the order in which they occurred and with statistically calculated center lines and upper and lower natural process limits. When data points fall outside of the calculated upper and lower natural process limits, they signal that the process is likely to have been influenced by nonrandom sources of variation, that is, that something special has taken place to produce remarkably high or low values.

core competencies for physicians The Accreditation Council for Graduate Medical Education (ACGME) has been in the vanguard of a movement in health professional education and maintenance of certification that focuses on educational outcomes relative to the acquisition of fundamental knowledge and skills. ACGME first established and endorsed the following core or general competencies for physicians in 1999: patient care, medical knowledge, practice-based learning and improvement, interpersonal and communication skills, professionalism, and systems-based practice.

customer The person or entity receiving the output or benefit of the output of a process. The customer could be a patient, a family, another department or unit, an insurer or payer, or an employer or purchaser of health care. Customers can be internal or external to an organization.

downstream and upstream A process can be viewed as a flow of steps and activities; just as a river flows and has a section that is upstream and a section that is downstream from a point of reference, a process can be viewed in a similar manner. Therefore, if one selects a particular step in a process, steps and activities that take place before this particular step can be referred to as being upstream, and steps and activities that happen after this same step can be referred to as downstream.

episode of care A period of use of the health care system for a patient with a problem or health condition, often related to the natural boundaries of the illness or condition. For example, an episode of care for a heart attack could cover emergency care, inpatient care, and related ambulatory and home care.

facilitator A person with skill and expertise in both clinical improvement and group process.

flowchart The graphic representation of a process.

huddle A short meeting of a clinical improvement team for check-in and reporting.

input The service or product a supplier provides to a process. For example, a grocery store might supply the inputs for a meal, a patient might supply a clinician with a new health problem, and a clinical laboratory might supply a clinician with the results of a diagnostic test.

mentor A person who has advanced skills in clinical improvement techniques, implementation, and evaluation and who shares that knowledge with a learner.

muda Japanese word for waste of effort or material in a process.

multivoting The group process decision-making technique that narrows down a long list of ideas to a small number of high-priority ideas. This is done by holding a straw vote to identify the ideas that are viewed as most and least promising and repeating straw votes and discussion to reduce the list to those that are determined to be the top priorities.

nominal group technique Idea-generation technique for group processes that develops ideas through input from individual group members.

output The service or product that a customer receives from a process. For example, the shopper at the grocery store might receive foods needed to prepare a meal, the clinician caring for a patient with a new problem might receive a chief complaint and a report on his or her history, and the clinician might receive a report from the clinical laboratory summarizing the diagnostic test results.

owner The person with the responsibility and authority to lead the improvement of a process. Also, the person with responsibility for a given process.

Pareto principle Named after the Italian economist, Wilfredo Pareto, the Pareto principle states that a few reasons account for the majority of variation. Sometimes referred to as the "80/20" rule: 80% of the variation is accounted for by 20% of the causes. When the Pareto principle is applied to improvement work, it often involves an effort to identify the "vital few" causes that most often account for the key result of interest.

pay for performance This is a method of health care reimbursement that aims to provide payments based on both the quality and cost of the care provided. This method of payment is in transition in the United States, but is generally going in the direction of what is called "value-based purchasing," which rewards organizations that deliver better quality at lower costs.

PDSA (Plan-Do-Study-Act) cycle A four-part method for discovering and correcting assignable causes to improve the quality of processes. The PDSA cycle represents the application of the scientific method for the purpose of improving work processes. A similar schema for continuous quality improvement related to a model of improvement was called Plan-Do-Check-Act (PDCA), originally developed by Walter Andrew Shewhart and popularized by W. Edwards Deming, who ascribed inherent variation in processes to chance (or random variation) and intermittent variation to assignable causes (or special cause variation).

process boundaries The points at which a process begins and ends.

process improvement An approach to understanding a process and to test change in it. Such efforts usually seek to reduce variation, improve benefit, and/or reduce cost for the person receiving benefit from the service or product produced by the process.

process variation Fluctuation in performance from time to time. This variation can be illustrated by the spread of data points that show the process output when graphically depicted over time using a run chart or a control chart.

purchaser A purchaser of health care, generally an employer or insurer or other payer, but also a patient or a family.

rank ordering The prioritizing technique that orders options from high to low based on decision-making criteria.

rework Work to redo or correct what was not done right the first time.

run chart Data display that shows data points in chronological order.

sponsor The leader in an organization who serves as an advocate for clinical improvement.

supplier The person, business, or other entity (such as another department, individual, or unit) responsible for an input to a process.

team leader The person identified to lead the clinical improvement team.

INDEX